The DeepFra...

A Structural Guide to Modern Facial Rejuvenation

An Anatomy-Driven Approach to Deep-Plane Facelift Surgery, Midface Elevation, and Neck Rejuvenation

BY ADAM LOWENSTEIN, MD

ISBN: 979-8-9943600-0-2

Adam Lowenstein
1722 State Street
Suite 101
Santa Barbara CA 93101
USA
https://sbplasticsurgeon.com

WHAT IS THE DEEPFRAME FACELIFT™?

The DeepFrame Facelift™ is a proprietary, anatomy-driven facial rejuvenation system created by Adam Lowenstein, MD, that restores youthful facial architecture by repositioning the deep structural layers of the face, rather than tightening the skin or adding artificial volume. It integrates true sub-periosteal midface elevation, multi-vector SMAS and platysma manipulation, and continuous deep-plane mobilization across the midface, lower face, jawline, and neck. By correcting aging at the level of the bone, deep fat compartments, ligaments, SMAS, and platysma, the DeepFrame Facelift™ is a deep plane facelift that re-establishes natural tissue relationships, preserves facial identity, and produces balanced, long-lasting results without fillers or fat grafting.

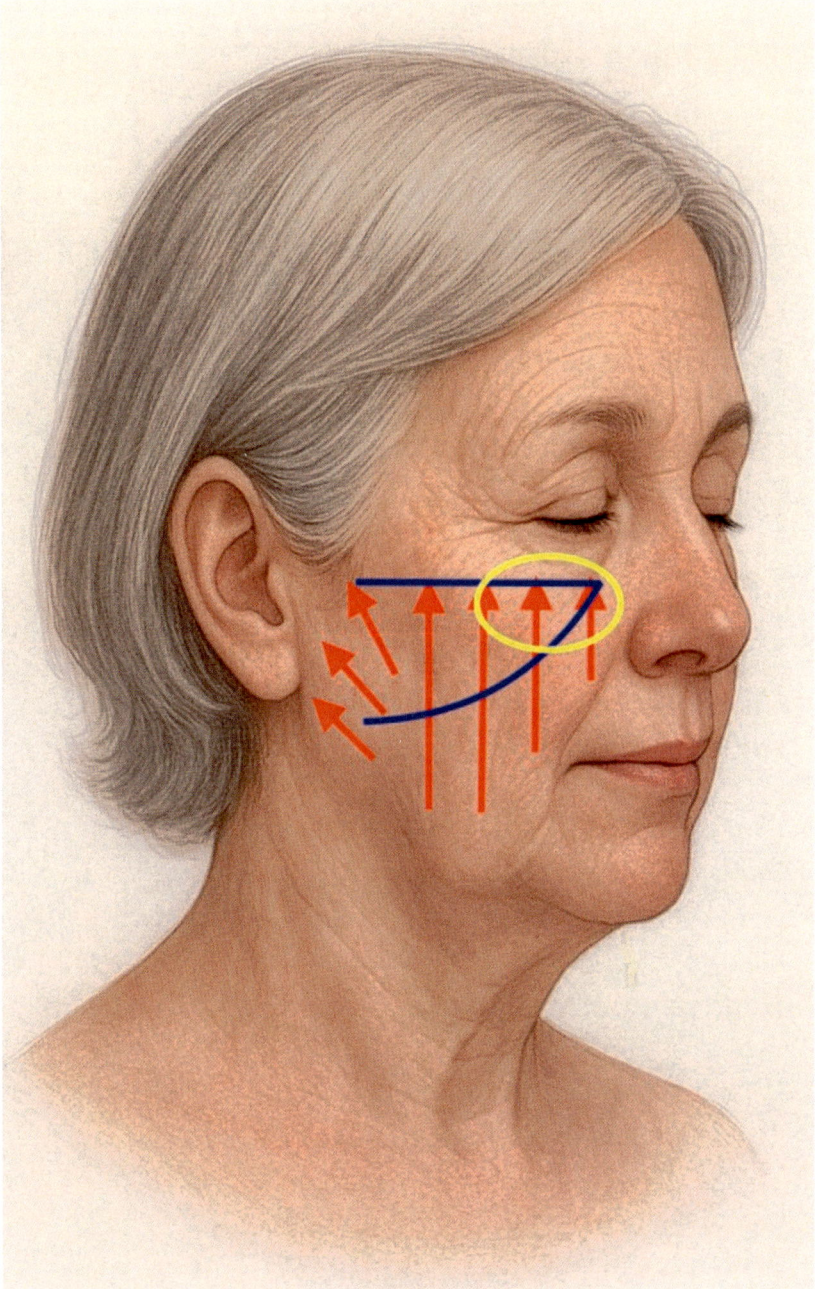

Adam Lowenstein, MD- The DeepFrame Facelift™

TABLE OF CONTENTS

INTRODUCTION

The DeepFrame Philosophy: A Comprehensive Structural System for Modern Facial Rejuvenation

Over the last half-century, facelift surgery has advanced through several conceptual eras: from the earliest skin-tightening procedures, to the introduction of SMAS manipulation, to the development of deep-plane approaches that sought to correct descent of deeper tissues. Despite this progress, many contemporary facelift techniques remain incomplete. They may focus on one anatomical layer, emphasize a single type of SMAS maneuver, or rely heavily on superficial tension to create the impression of lift. As a result, outcomes often fail to restore the full structural harmony of a youthful face, and longevity remains limited when foundational relationships are not corrected.

The DeepFrame Facelift™ was developed to address these limitations through a fully integrated, anatomy-driven system. It recognizes that aging is a three-dimensional, multi-vectorial process involving bone remodeling, deep fat descent, SMAS elongation, midface ptosis, and neck structural changes. Rather than approaching each region with isolated techniques, DeepFrame treats the face as a unified biomechanical structure in which individual components- midface, lower face, jawline, and neck- must be repositioned in relation to one another. By doing so, DeepFrame restores the natural tension lines, curvature, shadow patterns, and proportional relationships that define a youthful and authentic appearance.

A Unified Structural System

While various facelift techniques claim to rejuvenate the face, most address only fragments of the aging process. Some lifts rely exclusively on SMAS plication; others perform sub-SMAS dissection that mobilizes the lower face but leaves the midface structurally unsupported. High-SMAS variations can improve cheek contour but often fail to integrate the neck. Composite techniques elevate the skin and SMAS together, limiting vector control and preventing true shaping. Even deep-plane methods that effectively release the lower face may not reposition midfacial fat compartments in their correct vectors or may neglect the cervical mechanism entirely.

These approaches share a common limitation: they lack a comprehensive view of facial aging as a connected, load-bearing system. Aging does not occur in isolated pockets. Descent of the midface increases weight on the lower face. Jowl formation disrupts jawline definition. Platysmal laxity compromises the cervical angle. The neck, in turn, affects the way the lower face drapes, and the lower face affects the submandibular profile. Every region influences the next. When a facelift technique treats these regions separately, or only partially, results may be temporarily pleasing but structurally incomplete.

DeepFrame was created to solve this problem by addressing the face in its entirety, restoring the architectural relationships that existed before aging disrupted them.

The Three Structural Planes of DeepFrame

At the heart of DeepFrame is the recognition that different regions of the face require different depths of dissection, each chosen to restore the specific anatomic unit that has aged. DeepFrame employs three distinct but interrelated planes, each contributing to the final structural outcome:

1. Sub-Periosteal Midface Elevation
One of the most defining components of DeepFrame is the elevation of the midface in the sub-periosteal plane. By lifting the cheek off the maxilla, the native prominence of the malar region is restored. This shortens the lower eyelid, and smooths the nasojugal and nasolabial transitions. This maneuver repositions the deep fat pads vertically rather than laterally, returning them to the

convexity characteristic of youth. It is a key step that distinguishes DeepFrame from the majority of modern facelifts, which often leave the midface mostly untreated or attempt to camouflage midface descent with fillers. Elevating the midface structurally also reduces downward pressure on the lower face, improving jowl correction and enhancing jawline refinement. It is also key to improving deep nasolabial folds.

2. SMAS Deep-Plane Mobilization

In the lower face, DeepFrame manipulates the SMAS and lateral platysma as a unit. This produces powerful mobility of the jowls, marionette region, and lower facial fat compartments. By lifting these tissues in their natural vectors, DeepFrame restores mandibular definition and redistributes soft tissue volume that has descended below the jawline. Because the movement occurs in the deeper layers, skin tension remains low, preventing the swept, over-tightened appearance that plagued earlier facelift methods. SMAS manipulation is performed via sub-SMAS dissection with SMASectomy or SMAS plication, depending on the patient's pre-existing facial structure and the requirements for optimal tissue sculpture.

3. Vector-Specific SMAS Elevation

Tension vectors are used as a sculptural technique at the SMAS to restore cheek convexity, refine mandibular contour, and reinforce deep-plane repositioning. This allows the surgeon to tailor the procedure to each patient's unique anatomy, adding support where tissues are thin, and folding or tightening selectively where volume or curvature must be restored. In this way, DeepFrame merges the mobility of deep-plane surgery with the finesse of SMAS contouring, creating harmonious, individualized outcomes without reliance on fat grafting or heavy volumization. While sub-SMAS elevation and segmental resection is needed in more full faces, SMAS plication may be the best maneuver in the thinner aging face to restore the appearance of youth. The DeepFrame facelift allows for individualization without dogmatic repetition across different facial structures.

Vector Architecture: Reestablishing Natural Directionality

DeepFrame's strength lies not only in its choice of planes but also in its attention to vector science. Facial aging is fundamentally vertical, with tissues descending downward and slightly medially over time. Traditional facelifts attempted to correct aging by pulling laterally, which often led to distortion around the jaw, mouth, and nasolabial area.

DeepFrame restores tissues in the directions that oppose true gravitational descent. The midface is elevated vertically; the lower face is lifted vertically with a tailored oblique component; the jawline is refined using gentle superolateral support; and the neck benefits from a blend of vertical and superolateral vectors. These vectors flow continuously across facial regions, preventing the abrupt transitions or contour irregularities that arise when techniques mix directional pulls without anatomical rationale. Differentials in vector length from medial to lateral allow for some redundancy of deep tissue in the medial cheek, providing volume and precluding the need for fillers. The result is a face that appears naturally supported- not repositioned against its will.

The DeepFrame Neck: Integral to the System, Not an Afterthought

DeepFrame treats the neck as an extension of the lower face rather than a separate problem to be managed superficially. Platysmal support is provided in superolateral vectors that reinforce jawline definition and re-establish the cervicomental angle.[18-20] SMAS cervical mobilization smooths submandibular fullness and reduces band prominence without depending on aggressive skin excision or liposuction alone. Because the midface has already been elevated vertically, the downward load on the neck is reduced, enhancing both the immediate result and long-term stability.

The DeepFrame neck is a structural reconstruction of the cervicofacial continuum.

Identity Preservation Through Structural Restoration

One of the most compelling features of DeepFrame is the way it preserves, and in many cases restores, a patient's natural facial identity. Patients often fear looking "different" after a facelift, and those fears are justified with techniques that rely heavily on skin traction or impose an exaggerated aesthetic ideal. DeepFrame avoids this by working entirely in the deeper structural layers, repositioning tissues to where they originally sat rather than creating artificial shapes or overly straightened contours.

Because DeepFrame respects the patient's skeletal proportions, fat distribution, and muscular dynamics, the postoperative face appears familiar. The goal is always to achieve a version of the patient that looks rested, healthier, and naturally younger; not altered or stylized. This psychological harmony is a central pillar of the DeepFrame philosophy.

Avoiding the Pitfalls of Overfilling

In recent years, the widespread use of fillers and fat grafting has created a new aesthetic problem: the overfilled, heavy, or distorted face. While volume restoration has a role in some aspects of facial rejuvenation, it cannot substitute for structural repositioning. DeepFrame avoids the pitfalls associated with filler distortion or long-term fat graft hypertrophy by relying primarily on the patient's own repositioned tissues. When the deep fat pads of the midface and lower face are restored to their anatomical positions, much of the perceived need for volumization disappears. This results in a lighter, more natural appearance without the risk of an overstuffed or puffy look.

Longevity: Restoring Structural Integrity for Durable Results

DeepFrame achieves longevity not by tightening tissues harder but by repositioning deep tissues into their structurally favorable, anatomically correct locations. Skin is allowed to redrape passively without bearing mechanical load.[8,14] Because gravitational vectors are addressed at their source, the midface, SMAS, and platysma, the results maintain form for a decade or more, depending on lifestyle and genetic factors. Studies consistently demonstrate superior longevity for deep-plane methods that reposition rather than tighten.[5,7] DeepFrame enhances this further through its multi-plane integration and neck support.

Comparison With Other Facelift Techniques

Many modern techniques offer pieces of what DeepFrame accomplishes but do not assemble them into a unified, anatomically coherent strategy.

SMAS-only approaches may improve the lower face but leave the midface unchanged. Deep-plane variations may elevate the lower face effectively but neglect shaping or vector finesse. High-SMAS techniques may address cheek descent but lack cervical integration. Composite lifts combine skin and SMAS movement in one layer, sacrificing vector control. Short-scar vertical methods may improve certain features but lack the power required for significant jowl or neck changes.

DeepFrame synthesizes the advantages of all these approaches while eliminating their weaknesses. It is intentionally designed to be complete- an entire philosophy rather than a procedural modification.

The DeepFrame Facelift™ stands as a comprehensive system of structural facial rejuvenation that unites advanced anatomical knowledge with refined surgical technique. Through sub-periosteal midface elevation, SMAS deep-plane mobilization, tailored SMAS elevation, an anatomically precise vector system, and thoughtful cervical integration, it restores the face as a cohesive unit- lifting, shaping, and supporting tissues in the directions and planes where youth naturally resides.

DeepFrame does not reinvent the face. It restores the face. It does not depend on tension. It depends on architecture. It does not disguise aging. It corrects its underlying structure.

In doing so, DeepFrame Facelift represents the modern standard of natural, long-lasting, anatomy-driven facial rejuvenation and an evolution toward a more thoughtful, structural, and patient-centered approach to the art and science of the facelift.

In the following chapters, The DeepFrame Facelift™ will be explored in more detail. Anatomy, surgical development, postoperative expectations, and other concepts are presented and supported to educate surgeons and patients about the advantages of a procedure that creates a natural-looking, rejuvenated deep-plane facelift result.

CHAPTER 1

The Anatomy of the Deep Tissues of the Face and the Deep Plane

A meaningful understanding of facial rejuvenation begins not at the surface of the skin, but within the deep anatomical framework that gives the face its form, stability, and expressive capacity. The visible features commonly associated with facial aging, including jowls, deepening nasolabial folds, hollowing of the midface, elongation of the lower eyelid, and loss of cervical definition, are frequently misunderstood as superficial problems. In reality, these changes represent the downstream consequences of structural alterations occurring across multiple anatomical layers. Bone, deep fat, fascia, ligaments, and muscle each undergo age-related transformation, and their cumulative interaction produces the external signs of aging that patients seek to correct.

Historically, facial rejuvenation strategies focused on what was most visible and accessible, namely the skin. Early facelift techniques were predicated on the assumption that aging was primarily a cutaneous phenomenon characterized by laxity and redundancy. Surgical correction therefore emphasized excision and redraping of the skin envelope, often applying lateral tension to achieve immediate smoothing. While such approaches could temporarily improve appearance, their long-term shortcomings were predictable. Skin is not designed to serve as a primary load-bearing structure. When placed under sustained tension, it stretches, scars widen, and the underlying forces driving descent remain unaddressed. Over time, the results deteriorate, often accentuating rather than concealing aging.

As anatomical understanding advanced, it became increasingly clear that surface changes were secondary manifestations of deeper structural failure. Facial aging is now understood as a three-dimensional, multi-layer process governed by predictable biological and mechanical principles. Appreciating these principles is essential for any rejuvenation strategy that aims to produce natural, durable results. The deep tissues of the face do not age independently. Instead, changes at one level influence behavior at adjacent levels, creating a cascade of structural alterations that ultimately reshape facial form.

At the foundation of this process lies the facial skeleton. The bones of the face provide the rigid framework upon which all soft tissues depend for projection, support, and spatial orientation. With aging, this framework undergoes gradual but significant remodeling.[4] The maxilla retrudes, reducing anterior projection in the midface. The infraorbital rim resorbs, diminishing support beneath the lower eyelid. The pyriform aperture widens, altering perinasal contours. The mandible loses angular definition along both the body and angle, weakening the structural boundary that defines the lower face and neck.

These skeletal changes rarely draw attention in isolation, yet their influence is profound. Soft tissues are suspended from and draped over the bony framework. When that framework recedes, the mechanical environment supporting those tissues becomes less stable. Even when skin quality and soft tissue volume remain relatively preserved, the loss of skeletal projection undermines support and predisposes tissues to gravitational descent. This phenomenon explains why many individuals experience an acceleration of facial aging in midlife despite minimal changes in skin texture or thickness. The problem is not the skin itself, but the platform beneath it.

Skeletal remodeling cannot be reversed through soft tissue manipulation alone. However, understanding its role is critical for interpreting the behavior of overlying tissues and for appreciating why superficial approaches fail to produce durable rejuvenation. The skeleton sets the stage upon which all other age-related changes unfold.

Above the skeleton lie the deep fat compartments, which play a central role in defining youthful facial contour. For many years, facial fat was conceptualized as a diffuse and relatively homogeneous layer that simply diminished with age. This view has been fundamentally revised. Anatomical studies have demonstrated that facial fat is organized into discrete compartments, each with specific boundaries, vascular supply, and biomechanical properties. These compartments do not behave uniformly, nor do they age in the same way.[4]

Of particular importance are the deep medial cheek fat and the suborbicularis oculi fat (SOOF). Together, these structures contribute to malar projection, support the lower eyelid, and create the smooth transition between the eyelid and cheek that characterizes youthful faces. Contrary to common belief, aging of the midface is not primarily a process of fat loss. In most patients, deep fat volume remains present well into later decades of life. The problem lies in displacement rather than depletion.[1,2]

As skeletal projection diminishes and ligamentous support attenuates, deep fat compartments lose their stable anchoring points. Gravity and repetitive facial motion gradually shift these compartments inferiorly and medially. This displacement alters facial topography in predictable ways. The malar eminence flattens as deep fat descends from its youthful position. The lid cheek junction lengthens as cheek support beneath the lower eyelid is lost. Fixed anatomical boundaries such as the nasolabial fold become more pronounced as mobile tissues migrate against regions of relative fixation.

These changes are often misinterpreted as volume deficiency, leading to strategies that emphasize filling rather than repositioning. Adding volume without restoring structural position increases tissue mass without correcting its spatial relationship to surrounding anatomy. Over time, this approach can exacerbate descent, distort facial proportions, and create an unnatural appearance. Recognizing displacement as the primary mechanism of midface aging is therefore essential for understanding why structural repositioning yields superior outcomes.

The behavior of deep fat compartments is closely regulated by the retaining ligaments of the face. These ligaments form a complex network of fibrous attachments that anchor soft tissues to the underlying skeleton. They define zones of mobility and fixation, allowing facial tissues to move dynamically while resisting gravitational descent. In youth, retaining ligaments maintain stable spatial relationships between tissues, preserving facial contours even during expression.

With aging, retaining ligaments undergo gradual elongation and loss of tensile strength.[6] Importantly, they do not typically rupture. Instead, they stretch, permitting increasing degrees of soft tissue mobility relative to fixed skeletal points. This process explains why facial folds deepen over time. The nasolabial fold, for example, represents a boundary between relatively fixed tissue and increasingly mobile tissue above it. As tissues descend, the contrast between these zones becomes more pronounced, creating the appearance of a deepening crease.

Attempts to efface such folds without addressing the deeper descent that creates them are inherently limited. Surface smoothing does not alter the underlying mechanical imbalance. As long as mobile tissues continue to descend against fixed boundaries, folds will recur. Understanding the role of retaining ligaments reframes these features not as isolated problems, but as visible markers of deeper structural change.

Interwoven with the retaining ligaments and deep fat compartments is the superficial musculoaponeurotic system, commonly referred to as the SMAS. The SMAS is a continuous fascial layer that invests the facial musculature, suspends fat compartments, and transmits mechanical forces across the face. Although often described as if composed of discrete regional segments, the SMAS is anatomically unified. Its thickness, orientation, and mechanical properties vary by region, but its continuity is fundamental to facial support.

In youth, the SMAS functions as an efficient load sharing structure. It distributes the weight of overlying soft tissues and transmits forces generated by facial expression. With age, the SMAS elongates and loses its ability to effectively suspend the tissues it supports.[5,7] This elongation is a central driver of lower face aging. As the SMAS lengthens, jowl tissue descends, mandibular definition softens, and tissue redistributes below the jawline.

Because the SMAS functions as a continuous system, its failure in one region affects adjacent regions.[5,14,24] Elongation in the lower face influences cervical contour. Midface descent increases inferior load on the SMAS, accelerating its attenuation. Treating the SMAS uniformly without accounting for regional variability ignores these dynamics and often produces inconsistent results. Effective rejuvenation requires a nuanced understanding of how the SMAS behaves differently across the face and how its failure contributes to region specific aging patterns.

Inferiorly, the SMAS transitions seamlessly into the platysma, forming what is best understood as a cervicofacial sling. This sling supports the lower face and neck, maintaining mandibular definition and a sharp cervicomental angle in youth. The platysma is not merely a superficial muscle, but an integral component of the facial support system. [5,8]

With aging, the platysma elongates, loses tone, and often separates medially. These changes permit descent of subcutaneous tissues and contribute to platysmal banding, loss of cervical definition, and blunting of the cervicomental angle. Because the platysma is anatomically continuous with the SMAS, changes in the neck influence the lower face and vice versa. Treating the neck as an isolated aesthetic unit without restoring this continuity disrupts facial harmony and predisposes to early recurrence of laxity.[18,20,25]

The concept of the deep plane arises from the recognition that meaningful rejuvenation requires access to the anatomical layers where aging originates. The term deep plane is widely used in facelift surgery, yet it is frequently misunderstood. Anatomically, there is no single deep plane. Instead, there are multiple potential planes of dissection beneath the skin, each corresponding to a different structural layer and each appropriate for addressing different age-related changes.

SMAS identification and manipulation allow mobilization of the lower face and neck as a cohesive unit, either through sub-SMAS dissection or by SMAS plication. Both techniques have their roles in addressing SMAS elongation and platysmal failure. Subperiosteal dissection permits release and elevation of the midface at its point of skeletal attachment, correcting deep fat displacement and restoring cheek support. Deeper planes provide greater mobility and more powerful correction, but they require greater anatomical precision and judgment.

The critical insight is that effective rejuvenation does not depend on selecting a single plane and applying it universally. Instead, it depends on matching the plane of correction to the depth at which aging originates in each region. Superficial problems require superficial solutions. Structural problems require structural solutions. Confusing the two leads to undercorrection, overcorrection, or instability.

Facial aging is therefore best understood as a structural process involving skeletal remodeling, displacement of deep fat compartments, attenuation of retaining ligaments, elongation of the SMAS, and failure of the cervicofacial sling. These changes precede and drive the visible manifestations of aging at the skin surface. Treating the surface without restoring the underlying framework addresses appearance but not cause.

The deep plane should thus be regarded not as a specific technique, but as a conceptual framework for addressing aging at its anatomical source.[7,8] It reflects a shift from surface manipulation to structural restoration, from tension to repositioning, and from temporary improvement to durable change. With this anatomical foundation established, subsequent chapters examine how a structural facelift system applies these principles in an integrated and region-specific manner, translating deep anatomical understanding into long-term aesthetic and functional outcomes.

CHAPTER 2

What Is the DeepFrame Facelift™ Conceptually?

A clear definition of the DeepFrame Facelift™ must begin with an acknowledgment of the complexity of facial aging itself. Facial aging is not a single event, nor is it driven by uniform changes across tissues. Instead, it reflects the cumulative interaction of skeletal remodeling, displacement of deep fat compartments, attenuation of retaining ligaments, elongation of the superficial musculoaponeurotic system, and progressive weakening of the cervicofacial sling. These processes unfold over time and alter the spatial relationships among tissues that once worked in concert to produce youthful facial structure.[3,4,5] The visible signs of aging are therefore not isolated defects but expressions of an evolving structural imbalance.

The DeepFrame Facelift™ was developed as a direct response to this reality. It does not attempt to simplify aging into a single problem or address it through a single maneuver. Instead, it represents a systems-based approach designed to restore the deep framework of the face by intervening at the anatomical levels where aging originates. Its objective is not merely to tighten or smooth the face, but to reestablish the relationships among bone, deep soft tissues, fascia, muscle, and skin that govern facial form, function, and long-term stability.

This distinction is fundamental. Many facelift techniques succeed in producing short-term improvement by altering surface appearance, yet fail to deliver durable results because they do not address the underlying structural changes that drive aging. The DeepFrame Facelift™ seeks to correct those structural changes directly. In doing so, it reframes facial rejuvenation as a process of restoration rather than camouflage.

Traditional descriptions of facelift surgery often focus on a single defining feature. Procedures are categorized by whether they emphasize skin tightening, SMAS plication, sub-SMAS dissection, or deep-plane mobilization. While such classifications are useful for academic discussion, they risk oversimplifying a biological process that is inherently multidimensional. No single anatomical layer accounts for all age-related changes, and no isolated maneuver can reliably correct them across patients.

The DeepFrame Facelift™ is therefore intentionally structured as a system rather than a fixed recipe. It integrates multiple depths of correction and multiple vectors of repositioning, each selected according to the specific anatomical problem being addressed. Where aging originates at the skeletal interface, particularly in the midface, subperiosteal elevation is employed to restore deep support. Where fascial elongation contributes to contour change in the lower face, targeted manipulation of the SMAS restores suspension. Where cervical aging reflects failure of the platysmal sling, correction is performed within a framework that restores continuity rather than treating the neck as an isolated aesthetic unit.

This modular design allows the procedure to be adapted to individual anatomy and aging patterns while maintaining a coherent structural philosophy. Rather than forcing all patients into a standardized technical sequence, the DeepFrame approach prioritizes diagnosis over technique. The surgeon assesses which layers have failed, how they have failed, and how those failures interact. Correction is then tailored accordingly, guided by anatomy rather than by adherence to a predefined operative script.

A defining principle of the DeepFrame Facelift™ is repositioning rather than tightening. This distinction is often misunderstood, yet it lies at the core of durable facial rejuvenation. Tightening implies resisting gravity at the surface, frequently through skin tension or superficial fascial shortening. While this can temporarily improve contour, it places sustained load on tissues that are not designed to bear it. Over time, these tissues stretch, scars widen, and the original imbalance reasserts itself.

Repositioning, by contrast, restores tissues toward their anatomically appropriate locations. When deep structures are returned closer to their youthful position, the forces acting upon them are fundamentally altered. Gravitational load is reduced at its source rather than resisted at the surface. This difference is biomechanical rather than semantic. It reflects an understanding of how tissues bear load, how they fail, and how they can be stabilized over time.

When tissues are repositioned at the level of bone, deep fat, and robust fascial structures, load is transferred to tissues capable of maintaining support. Skin is relieved of its role as a structural element and can function as a covering rather than as a suspension system. The DeepFrame Facelift™ therefore emphasizes restoration of position rather than compensation through tension. This approach aligns with the biological behavior of facial tissues and underpins the longevity of its results.

Another defining feature of the DeepFrame Facelift™ is its treatment of the face and neck as a unified anatomical system. Facial regions do not age independently. Descent of the midface increases the inferior load on the lower face. Elongation of the SMAS influences both jowl formation and cervical contour. Failure of the platysmal sling undermines mandibular definition and blunts the cervicomental angle. These processes interact continuously, and attempts to correct one region in isolation often destabilize adjacent regions.

The DeepFrame approach addresses this interdependence directly. Correction in one region is planned to reinforce, rather than oppose, correction in adjacent regions. Vector planning is coordinated across the midface, lower face, and neck to ensure that forces are harmonized rather than competing. This integration distinguishes structural rejuvenation from fragmented approaches that treat aesthetic units in isolation and contributes to both aesthetic coherence and mechanical stability.[8][14]

Skin management within the DeepFrame Facelift™ follows from this structural philosophy. Skin is not used as a primary support structure. Instead, it is redraped passively over a restored framework of deep tissues. Because deep support has been reestablished, skin can conform naturally without being placed under significant tension. This has important implications for both appearance and safety.

Low tension skin redraping improves scar quality by reducing stress across closures. It preserves vascular supply by avoiding excessive undermining and tension. It reduces the risk of a pulled or operated appearance by allowing surface contours to reflect underlying anatomy rather than imposed force. In this context, skin redraping is a consequence of structural correction rather than its mechanism. This inversion of priorities is central to the DeepFrame philosophy.

Preservation of facial identity is another core objective of the DeepFrame Facelift™. Patients rarely seek to look like a different person. Rather, they seek to look like themselves at an earlier point in time. Techniques that rely on uniform vectors, excessive tightening, or volumetric exaggeration risk overriding individual anatomy and producing a generic or artificial result.

By restoring tissues toward their pre-aging anatomical positions, the DeepFrame approach respects each patient's inherent skeletal structure, soft tissue distribution, and expressive patterns. Correction follows anatomy rather than imposing an external aesthetic template. This allows for significant rejuvenation while preserving recognizability. Facial expression remains natural because muscles are not restricted by surface tension or distorted by misplaced volume.

An important conceptual distinction within the DeepFrame Facelift™ is the idea of a structural reset rather than an attempt to arrest aging. Aging is a continuous biological process driven by genetics, environment, and time. It cannot be halted surgically. Attempts to promise permanence are therefore misleading and set unrealistic expectations.

Instead, the DeepFrame Facelift™ establishes a new anatomical baseline by correcting the cumulative structural distortions that have developed over years or decades. From this reset point, aging resumes in a more favorable configuration. Changes occur more slowly and proportionately, and facial harmony is preserved for a longer period. This perspective shapes both surgical planning and patient counseling. The emphasis is placed on durability, balance, and realism rather than on the illusion of permanence.

Because the DeepFrame Facelift™ is a systems based approach rather than a standardized procedure, its success depends heavily on surgical judgment. The surgeon must evaluate which layers require correction, which vectors are appropriate, and how aggressively each component should be applied. This decision-making process is guided by anatomy, tissue quality, and aging pattern rather than by rigid adherence to a protocol.

This reliance on judgment resists commoditization. It underscores the importance of anatomical expertise, experience, and restraint. The DeepFrame approach provides a framework for decision-making, not a formula to be applied uniformly. Its effectiveness lies in its adaptability, allowing the surgeon to respond to the unique structural needs of each face.

In summary, the DeepFrame Facelift™ is an anatomy-driven, systems-based approach to facial rejuvenation that restores the deep structural framework of the aging face. By integrating subperiosteal midface elevation, region-specific manipulation of the SMAS, coordinated cervical support, and low-tension skin redraping, it addresses aging at its anatomical source rather than compensating for its surface manifestations.

This structural philosophy establishes the conditions necessary for natural appearance, mechanical stability, and long term durability. With this framework defined, the following chapter examines the vectors of correction that guide tissue repositioning and play a critical role in determining both aesthetic outcome and longevity.

CHAPTER 3

The Vectors of the DeepFrame Facelift™

Among all elements of facelift surgery, vector planning is among the most consequential and the most frequently misunderstood. Discussions of facial rejuvenation often focus on planes of dissection, layers of manipulation, or named techniques, yet these considerations alone do not determine outcome. Vectors describe both direction and magnitude. It is the direction, magnitude, and integration of corrective forces applied to facial tissues that ultimately govern both aesthetic result and long-term stability. Vectors represent the functional expression of surgical philosophy. They translate anatomical understanding into mechanical action.

Facial aging unfolds along predictable directions dictated by gravity, skeletal architecture, ligamentous support, and the mechanical properties of soft tissues.[3,8] When rejuvenation strategies ignore these vectors or attempt to oppose them superficially, results may appear improved in the short term but rarely endure. Effective facial rejuvenation requires correction along the same

Figure 1

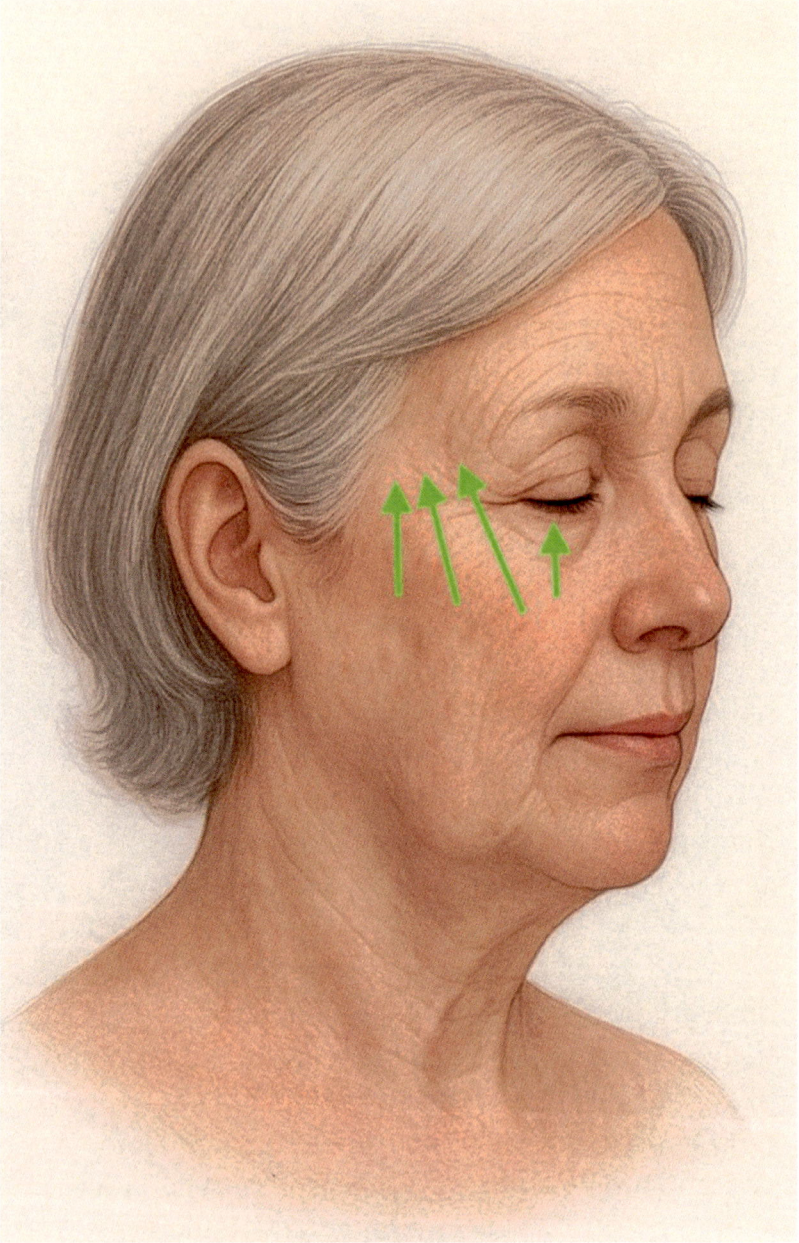

Vectors of Midface Elevation

directional paths through which aging occurred, applied at the depth where structural failure originated. This principle lies at the core of the DeepFrame Facelift™.

The DeepFrame approach is distinguished not by the application of force alone, but by how that force is conceived and distributed. Vector planning is anatomically driven, region-specific, and structurally integrated. Rather than applying uniform traction across the face, the DeepFrame Facelift™ restores tissues along vectors that mirror their original descent and respect the biomechanical behavior of each anatomical layer. This alignment between aging vectors and corrective vectors is central to achieving natural appearance, functional preservation, and durability.

Facial aging is not random. It reflects the cumulative effect of gravitational forces acting on tissues whose support systems have progressively weakened. Skeletal remodeling reduces projection. Retaining ligaments elongate. Fascial structures lose tensile efficiency. As these changes occur, soft tissues respond by migrating along paths of least resistance. These paths are remarkably consistent across patients, even though the pace and degree of aging vary individually.

In the midface, aging is predominantly vertical. [2,4,10] Deep fat compartments and overlying soft tissues descend inferiorly away from the orbit as

Figure 2

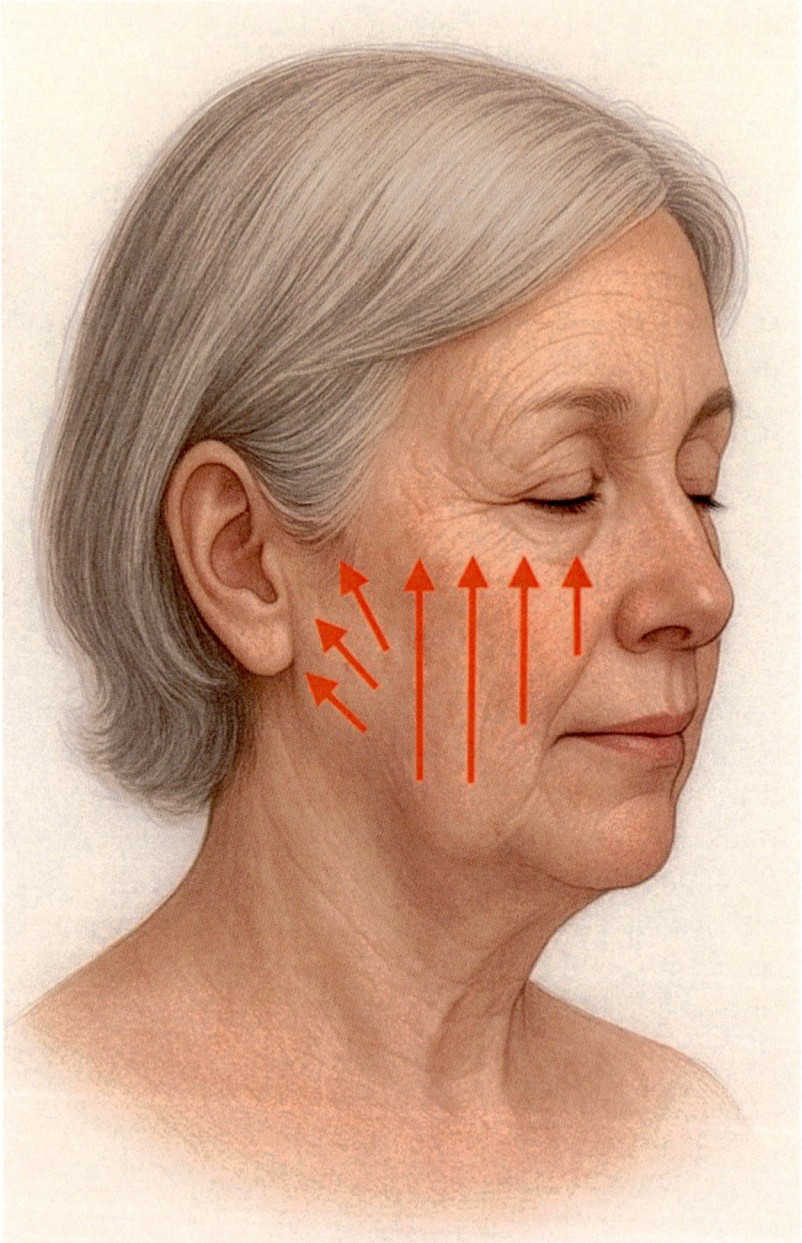

Vectors of SMAS Elevation

skeletal support diminishes and ligamentous resistance attenuates. This vertical descent lengthens the lower eyelid, flattens the malar eminence, and creates the appearance of hollowing despite preserved volume. In the lower face, aging follows a combined vertical and inferomedial trajectory. As the SMAS elongates, jowl tissue descends downward and inward, blunting the mandibular border and altering oral commissure position. Some surgeons simplify this as "rotational" laxity, rather than treating different vectors of descent in individualized manners. In the neck, aging proceeds along inferior and anterior vectors as the platysmal sling weakens and cervical support fails.

These directional patterns are not arbitrary. They reflect the orientation of skeletal surfaces, the arrangement of ligaments, and the mechanical behavior of fascia under load. When corrective forces are applied without regard to these natural vectors, tissues are displaced along unnatural paths. This mismatch between aging vectors and corrective vectors produces inefficiency, distortion, and early relapse. Understanding aging as a vector-based process is, therefore, foundational to durable rejuvenation.

The midface provides the clearest illustration of this principle. Midfacial aging is driven primarily by vertical descent of deep tissues relative to the orbit. Attempts to rejuvenate the midface through

Figure 3

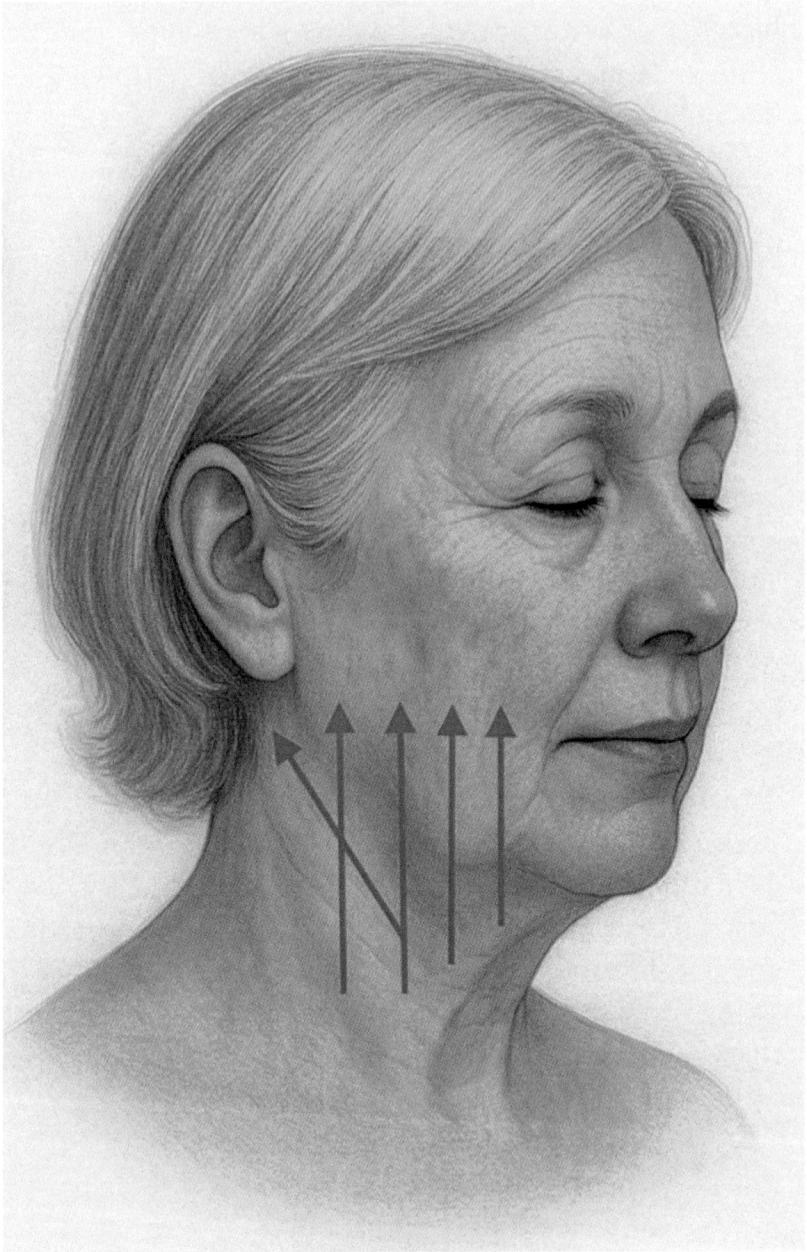

Vectors of Neck Elevation

lateral traction, whether via skin tightening or lateral SMAS pull, fail to restore malar height and often exacerbate facial flattening. Lateral vectors do not counteract vertical descent.[7,9] Instead, they redirect tissues sideways, stretching them across fixed anatomical boundaries without restoring their original position.

The DeepFrame Facelift™ addresses midface aging through vertical and superolateral vectors applied at the level of skeletal attachment. (Figure 1) Subperiosteal elevation allows the cheek to be mobilized as a unit and repositioned upward beneath the orbit. This correction restores the deep fat compartments to a position closer to their youthful location, reestablishing malar projection and lower eyelid support. Because the vector of correction mirrors the vector of descent, less force is required to achieve meaningful improvement.

This alignment has important biomechanical consequences. When tissues are repositioned along their original path of descent, resistance is minimized and fixation is more stable. The restored midface also reduces inferior load transmitted to the lower face and neck. In this way, vertical midface correction functions not only as a localized improvement but as a foundational maneuver that stabilizes the entire facial support system.

The lower face presents a more complex vector environment. Aging in this region does not occur along a single axis. Jowl formation reflects both vertical descent and medial migration of soft tissues as SMAS support weakens and mandibular projection diminishes.[19,21,22] Effective correction, therefore, requires composite vectors that address both components of movement.[9,14]

The DeepFrame Facelift™ applies these composite vectors through region-specific manipulation of the SMAS. (Figure 2) Vertical support restores suspension and repositions jowl tissue superiorly into the cheek. Oblique lateral refinement sharpens mandibular definition without redirecting tissues unnaturally toward the ear. This balance is critical. Excessive lateral traction risks widening the lower face, distorting the oral commissure, and producing a pulled appearance. Insufficient vertical support fails to counteract gravitational descent and leads to early recurrence.

By integrating vertical and oblique components, the DeepFrame approach restores lower face contour while preserving facial proportions and expression. The goal is not to move tissues laterally, but to reestablish their vertical position and refine their boundary against the mandible. This distinction differentiates structural correction from techniques that rely primarily on lateral pull.

Vector planning within the DeepFrame Facelift™ extends beyond individual regions to encompass the face and neck as a unified

44

biomechanical system. Facial regions do not exist in isolation. A correction in one area inevitably alters force distribution elsewhere. When midface elevation is achieved, inferior forces acting on the lower face are reduced. When lower face support is restored, strain on the platysma diminishes. Conversely, when these relationships are ignored, corrective forces may compete rather than reinforce one another.

The DeepFrame approach emphasizes continuity of vectors across regions. Vector planning is coordinated so that forces applied in the midface, lower face, and neck are complementary. This integration distributes load across deeper support structures and avoids the creation of stress concentrations that predispose to relapse. Fragmented vector planning, in contrast, produces instability. A tightly pulled neck beneath an unsupported jawline, or a laterally tightened face beneath a descended midface, reflects competing vectors rather than harmonious correction.

Neck aging progresses in an inferior and medial direction, and the DeepFrame technique addresses this in multiple ways. As the platysma in the neck is an extension of the SMAS in the face, the inferior displacement of the SMAS with aging compounds tissue excess below the mandible. As the base of the sling, the tissue excess has nowhere to go and becomes redundant.

Vertical SMAS elevation consistently improves the neck, and a patient concerned about neck redundancy can always see improvement in a mirror when the surgeon demonstrates superior SMAS correction alone. Lateral traction on the neck following SMAS manipulation helps rejuvenate the neck, counteracting the medial pull of the platysma over time. (Figure 3) If tight platysmal bands additionally need to be addressed, a platysmaplasty is used to further define the cervicomental angle. Many patients prefer to avoid the platysmaplasty as the severity of the cervicomental angle can produce an operated appearance, and this should be addressed with the patient during the planning stages of the procedure.

Depth and vector are inseparable considerations. A vector applied at the wrong depth is inherently inefficient.[8,14] Superficial vectors applied at the level of the skin require greater force to achieve visible change. Because skin and superficial tissues are not designed to bear sustained load, these corrections are prone to stretch and relapse. In addition, superficial traction often distorts surface anatomy by pulling tissues across fixed landmarks.

The DeepFrame Facelift™ applies vectors at the depth appropriate to the anatomical problem being addressed. Vertical midface vectors (Figure 1) are applied subperiosteally at the skeletal interface, where deep fat compartments can be mobilized and repositioned effectively. Lower face vectors (Figure

2) are applied through the SMAS, which is capable of transmitting force and maintaining suspension. Cervical vectors (Figure 3) are coordinated through the platysma and deeper neck structures to restore sling integrity rather than relying on skin tension.

This alignment of depth and direction allows correction to be achieved with minimal force and maximal stability. When tissues are repositioned at depth, skin redrapes passively and naturally. Surface appearance reflects restored structure rather than imposed tension. This principle underlies both the natural look and the durability associated with structural rejuvenation.

A common source of unnatural results in facelift surgery is the application of uniform vectors across the face. Faces are not symmetrical mechanical systems, and aging does not affect all regions equally. Applying the same direction and magnitude of force everywhere ignores regional differences in anatomy, tissue quality, and aging pattern. Uniform vector application often produces overcorrection in some areas and undercorrection in others, resulting in imbalance and distortion.

The DeepFrame Facelift™ avoids this error by tailoring vectors to each region while maintaining overall coherence. Midface vectors differ from lower face vectors, which differ from cervical vectors. Yet these regional corrections are unified by a common structural philosophy and coordinated planning. This approach allows meaningful rejuvenation without imposing a standardized aesthetic or altering individual facial character.

Dynamic considerations further distinguish effective vector planning from superficial traction. Facial tissues must move naturally during expression, speech, mastication, and swallowing. Vectors that overly constrain movement or redirect muscular forces can produce stiffness, asymmetry, or distortion during animation. These effects may be subtle at rest but become evident during expression.

By restoring tissues along anatomically appropriate vectors and placing support in deep layers, the DeepFrame approach preserves dynamic function. Muscles operate within restored anatomical boundaries rather than against surface tension. Expression remains fluid because the forces governing movement have not been altered artificially. This preservation of function contributes significantly to patient satisfaction, even when it is not consciously articulated.

Longevity in facelift surgery is closely linked to biomechanical efficiency. Corrections that align with natural aging vectors require less sustained force and place less stress on fixation points. As a result, they maintain their effect longer and age more gracefully. Techniques that rely on resisting gravity through tension must continually oppose forces that have not been altered at their source. Over time, such resistance fails.

The DeepFrame Facelift™ achieves longevity not by attempting to resist aging, but by restoring anatomy so that aging resumes from a corrected and mechanically favorable baseline. When tissues are repositioned along their original vectors of descent and supported at depth, subsequent aging occurs more slowly and proportionately. The face does not appear frozen in time, but it maintains harmony and balance as changes unfold.

Vectors, therefore, represent more than technical choices. They embody the underlying philosophy of facial rejuvenation. When correction follows the same paths along which aging occurred, results are more natural, more stable, and more durable. When vectors are misaligned, even technically precise surgery may fail to deliver lasting benefit.

The DeepFrame Facelift™ employs region-specific, anatomically aligned vectors applied at appropriate depths to restore facial architecture as an integrated system. This approach minimizes distortion, preserves expression, and establishes the biomechanical foundation upon which long term rejuvenation depends. In the chapters that follow, this vector based philosophy is applied to specific facial regions, illustrating how structural principles translate into consistent and durable clinical outcomes.

CHAPTER 4

How the DeepFrame Facelift™ Addresses the Eyes

The periorbital region occupies a unique position in facial aesthetics. It is both anatomically intricate and visually dominant, and even subtle alterations in contour, support, or proportion can dramatically influence perceived age, vitality, and emotional state. Patients frequently describe appearing tired, sad, or unwell despite feeling energetic and healthy. These impressions are rarely explained by eyelid skin changes alone. Instead, they reflect deeper structural alterations involving the orbit, the midface, and the complex soft tissue relationships that support the eyelids.

A central premise of the DeepFrame Facelift™ is that the eyes cannot be treated as an isolated aesthetic unit. The lower eyelid does not exist independently of the cheek, nor does its position depend solely on the quality of its skin. The appearance and function of the eyelid are inseparably linked to the integrity of midface support, the projection of the infraorbital skeleton, the behavior of deep fat compartments, and the mechanics of the orbicularis oculi muscle.[2,12] Meaningful periorbital rejuvenation, therefore, requires a structural approach that addresses these relationships rather than focusing narrowly on the eyelid surface.

With aging, the upper eyelid undergoes predictable structural and soft-tissue changes that alter both appearance and function. Progressive skin laxity leads to dermatochalasis, while attenuation of the orbital septum allows preaponeurotic fat to bulge or descend. At the same time, loss of brow support and subtle bony remodeling of the superior orbital rim reduce upper eyelid show and contribute to a heavier, more tired look. These changes are often compounded by weakening of the levator aponeurosis, which can lower the eyelid margin and further obscure the natural lid crease, emphasizing fatigue and age.

In youth, the lower eyelid and cheek form a continuous anatomical unit.[12,13] The lid cheek junction is short, smooth, and gently convex. There is no visible step off, hollow, or shadow separating the eyelid from the cheek. The cheek provides a stable and supportive platform beneath the eyelid, allowing the lid to maintain appropriate tone, contour, and position without reliance on skin tension. This relationship is central to a rested and healthy appearance.

With aging, this integrated structure progressively deteriorates. Skeletal remodeling of the maxilla and infraorbital rim reduces anterior projection beneath the orbit. Retaining ligaments attenuate and lose resistance to gravitational forces. Deep midface fat compartments descend vertically away from the orbit. As these changes accumulate, the cheek migrates inferiorly and posteriorly relative to the lower eyelid.

This structural shift produces the hallmark features of periorbital aging. The lower eyelid appears elongated as the cheek descends away from it. A hollow or shadow develops at the lid cheek junction, often described as a tear trough deformity. The transition between eyelid and cheek becomes abrupt rather than smooth. Importantly, these changes occur even in patients with relatively good eyelid skin quality and minimal surface laxity. They reflect loss of support rather than excess tissue.

When this distinction is not recognized, periorbital rejuvenation strategies often focus on the eyelid itself. Skin excision, skin tightening, or isolated removal of orbital fat may temporarily improve appearance, but they do not address the underlying structural failure. In many cases, they exacerbate it. Removing tissue from an already unsupported eyelid can further destabilize its position and compromise function.[12,13] Over time, such approaches frequently lead to recurrent deformity or new problems that are more difficult to correct.

The DeepFrame Facelift™ approaches the periorbital region from a fundamentally different perspective. Rather than asking how to modify the eyelid, it asks why the eyelid appears aged in the first place. In the majority of patients, the answer lies not in the lower eyelid itself but in the midface beneath it. Restoring periorbital youthfulness, therefore, begins with restoring midface position and support.

The upper eyelid skin excess that accompanies aging is commonly addressed with simple excision. Removing the redundancy that this skin represents allows visualization of the nuances of the upper orbit. Addressing brow position, if required, should be done prior to upper lid procedures to avoid over resection of upper lid skin.

During the upper lid component of the DeepFrame Facelift™, the lateral skin excision is deepened to expose the temporalis fascia and the lateral orbit. This region serves as the anchor point for the midface lift. The sub-periosteal dissection of the midface begins here, extending toward the lateral aspect of the inferior orbital rim, allowing release of the inferior orbicularis and overlying soft tissues of the cheek.

The most powerful periorbital effect of the DeepFrame Facelift™ arises from subperiosteal midface elevation. By releasing the midface at its skeletal attachment, the cheek can be mobilized as a structural unit and repositioned superiorly and anteriorly beneath the orbit. This maneuver restores the anatomical buttress that supports the lower eyelid complex.[10,11]. The subperiosteal release of the midface soft tissue is performed through the lateral aspect of the subciliary incision, while the skin overlying the orbicularis is lifted and redundancy removed as the soft tissue is suspended.

As the cheek returns toward its youthful position relative to the orbit, several changes occur simultaneously. The lid cheek junction shortens as the cheek rises to meet the eyelid. The hollow at this junction diminishes because the underlying platform has been restored rather than filled. The contour of the lower eyelid appears smoother and more continuous with the cheek. These improvements occur without placing tension on eyelid skin and without introducing foreign or added volume.

Because correction is achieved at the depth where aging originates, the result is mechanically stable. The repositioned cheek supports the eyelid passively, reducing the forces that would otherwise act to elongate or distort it over time. This structural correction addresses the cause of periorbital aging rather than its surface manifestations.

The orbicularis oculi muscle plays a central role in eyelid function and appearance. It is responsible

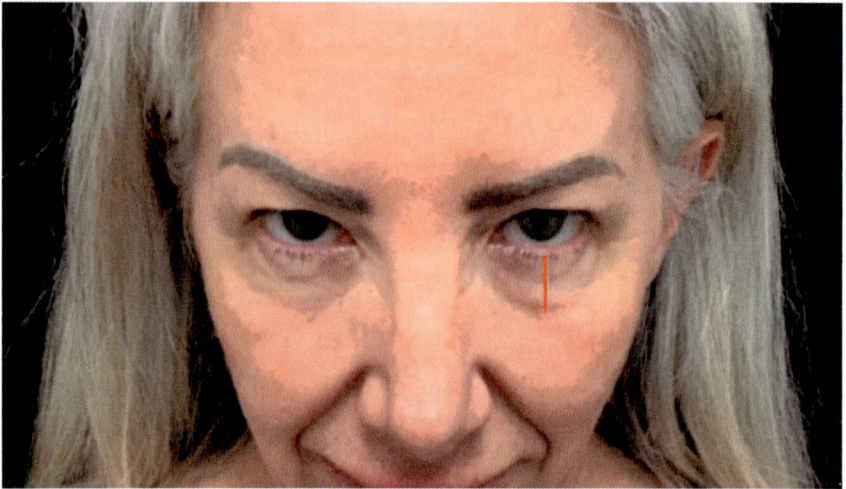

Shortening of the lower lid with The DeepFrame Facelift™. The red line indicates lower lid length, improved following blepharoplasty and deep plane midface elevation.

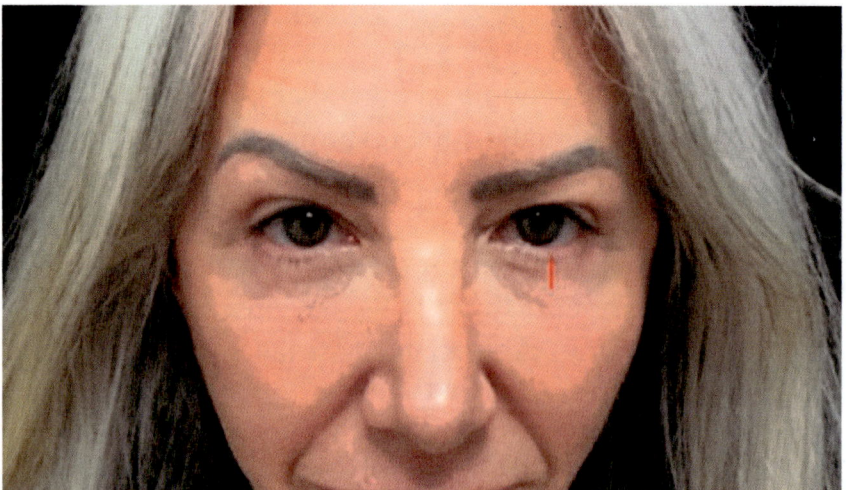

for blinking, eyelid tone, and subtle expressive movements. In youth, the orbicularis functions within a balanced mechanical environment supported by the cheek beneath it and constrained by intact ligamentous attachments. With aging and midface descent, this balance is disrupted.

Loss of cheek support allows elongation and inferior displacement of the orbicularis complex. This contributes to eyelid laxity, pseudo-herniation of orbital fat, and irregular contour during expression. Superficial tightening of eyelid skin may temporarily mask these changes, but it does not restore normal mechanics. In some cases, it increases stress on the orbicularis and exacerbates functional problems such as dryness or incomplete closure.

By repositioning the cheek beneath the eyelid, the DeepFrame Facelift™ improves orbicularis support indirectly. The muscle is allowed to function within a restored anatomical framework rather than being constrained by surface tension. Blink mechanics are preserved. Eyelid tone improves as structural support is reestablished. This indirect restoration of function is a critical advantage of structural periorbital rejuvenation.

When adjunctive eyelid procedures are indicated, they can be performed more conservatively within this restored environment. Skin excision can be minimized. Fat manipulation can be restrained. The risk of overcorrection is reduced because the eyelid no longer bears the burden of compensating for midface descent. In this way, the DeepFrame approach enhances both the safety and effectiveness of ancillary eyelid surgery.

The lid cheek junction itself deserves particular attention. It is one of the most important aesthetic landmarks of the face and a powerful indicator of age. Lengthening of this junction is among the earliest and most reliable signs of periorbital aging. Yet it is also one of the most commonly misinterpreted features.

True shortening of the lid cheek junction cannot be achieved by tightening the eyelid. Removing skin may elevate the lid margin temporarily, but it does not restore the cheek beneath it. The apparent improvement is often short-lived and may compromise eyelid position. Structural rejuvenation of the lid cheek junction depends on elevating the cheek rather than manipulating the eyelid.

The DeepFrame Facelift™ achieves this by reestablishing the original spatial relationship between the eyelid and midface. As the cheek is restored to its proper height, the lid cheek junction shortens naturally. The transition becomes smooth and continuous, reflecting restored anatomy rather than surgical artifice.

Another frequent source of periorbital distortion arises from volumetric camouflage. Fillers and fat grafting are commonly used to soften hollows at the lid cheek junction. While they may temporarily reduce shadowing, they do not correct cheek descent. Over time, added volume often migrates, attracts edema, or interferes with eyelid dynamics. The periorbital region is particularly sensitive to these effects, and even small irregularities are readily apparent.

Fat grafting introduces additional variability related to survival and potential hypertrophy. In a region where millimeters matter, unpredictability is poorly tolerated. Moreover, adding volume to an unsupported eyelid cheek complex increases mass without restoring support, potentially accelerating further descent.

By restoring native tissue position, the DeepFrame Facelift™ reduces reliance on volumetric camouflage. When true volume deficiency exists, it can be addressed selectively and conservatively within a structurally corrected framework. This sequencing is critical. Volume should refine restored anatomy, not attempt to substitute for it.

Preservation of expression and identity is particularly important in the periorbital region. The eyes are central to emotional communication, and even subtle distortion is immediately perceived.

Overcorrection, excessive tightening, or inappropriate volumization can produce a startled, hollow, or artificial appearance that undermines patient satisfaction regardless of technical success.

Structural periorbital rejuvenation prioritizes preservation of blink mechanics, ocular comfort, and expressive nuance. Because the DeepFrame approach minimizes direct manipulation of eyelid skin and avoids excessive tension, it improves appearance while maintaining functional integrity. Patients appear more rested and alert, not altered. This distinction is often difficult to quantify but immediately recognizable.

Periorbital rejuvenation also cannot be considered in isolation from the rest of the face. Changes in midface position influence eyelid support. Lower face and neck correction alter global facial balance. Treating these regions independently often produces discordant results, such as youthful eyes above an aged midface or an elevated cheek beneath an untreated neck.

The DeepFrame Facelift™ integrates periorbital correction into a comprehensive facial strategy. Midface elevation supports the eyes. Lower face and cervical correction restore harmony across regions. This integration ensures that improvements around the eyes are consistent with changes elsewhere on the face, reinforcing a cohesive and natural result.

Periorbital aging is therefore best understood as a structural problem driven by midface descent, skeletal remodeling, and loss of deep support beneath the lower eyelid. Superficial treatments that focus on eyelid skin or volume alone fail to address these underlying causes and frequently produce limited or unstable outcomes.

The DeepFrame Facelift™ addresses the eyes by restoring the anatomical relationship between the cheek and orbit through subperiosteal midface elevation. This structural correction shortens the lid cheek junction, smooths contour, preserves function, and produces natural, durable rejuvenation that respects both anatomy and identity. By treating the eyes as part of an integrated facial framework rather than as an isolated unit, it achieves results that are both aesthetically refined and mechanically sound.

CHAPTER 4A

Common Errors When the Eyes Are Treated Superficially

Errors in periorbital rejuvenation arise most often from misunderstanding the structural basis of aging around the eyes. Because changes in this region are visually prominent and emotionally charged, there is a strong temptation to intervene directly at the level of the eyelid. While such approaches may produce short-term visual improvement, they frequently fail to address the anatomical forces responsible for the aged appearance. Over time, these errors contribute to distortion, dissatisfaction, and the need for repeated or escalating intervention.

One of the most common mistakes is treating the lower eyelid as an isolated aesthetic unit. Skin excision, tightening, resurfacing, or fat manipulation may temporarily improve surface appearance, but without restoration of midface support the eyelid remains structurally compromised. The lower eyelid depends on the cheek for mechanical support. When the cheek has descended away from the orbit, the eyelid is subjected to forces it cannot resist indefinitely. As a result, superficial eyelid treatments often lead to recurrent hollowing, elongation of the lid cheek junction, or progressive laxity despite initial improvement.

A closely related error is misinterpreting displacement as volume loss. Hollows beneath the eyes are frequently assumed to represent a deficiency of tissue rather than the migration of tissue away from its youthful position.[12,16] This assumption drives the use of fillers or fat grafting in the tear trough region without correcting the underlying cause of the hollow. When volume is added to a region that has lost structural support, weight increases without restoring architecture. Over time, this may worsen edema, create contour irregularities, or interfere with eyelid dynamics. The appearance may become fuller without becoming younger, and repeated treatments are often required to maintain the illusion of correction.

Excessive reliance on fillers near the orbit represents another frequent pitfall. The periorbital region has limited tolerance for injected material. Skin is thin, lymphatic drainage is delicate, and even small volume changes can be visually apparent. Fillers placed beneath the lower eyelid may migrate, attract fluid, or become visible as contour irregularities. Even when expertly placed, they do not restore the position of the cheek relative to the orbit. Over time, repeated filler use often produces a puffy or amorphous appearance that blunts natural transitions and complicates future surgical correction.[16,17]

Over-tightening of eyelid skin is another common error rooted in surface-level thinking. Attempts to rejuvenate the eyes by tightening skin alone do not restore deep support and place stress on tissues not designed to bear sustained load. This approach may produce a pulled, hollowed, or fatigued appearance and can interfere with normal eyelid closure. Functional complications such as dryness or irritation may follow, particularly when eyelid tightening is performed in the absence of midface correction. Even when complications are avoided, the aesthetic result often deteriorates as underlying structural forces continue to act.

Perhaps the most fundamental error in superficial periorbital treatment is failure to integrate eyelid planning with midface correction. The appearance of the eyes is inseparable from cheek position, skeletal projection, and global facial balance. Treating the eyelids independently may improve one feature while leaving adjacent regions discordant. Youthful appearing eyes above a descended midface often look unnatural and unstable. Conversely, attempts to correct the eyelids aggressively in isolation can exaggerate imbalance elsewhere on the face.

Fragmented planning reflects a conceptual error rather than a technical one. When periorbital aging is viewed as a surface problem, solutions are directed toward the surface. When it is understood as a structural problem, correction shifts toward restoring support beneath the eyelid. Structural approaches such as the DeepFrame Facelift™ avoid these errors by addressing the relationships that govern eyelid position and contour rather than focusing narrowly on eyelid appearance.

Superficial treatment of periorbital aging can produce transient improvement, but it often does so at the cost of long-term instability. Errors arise when displacement is mistaken for deficiency and when eyelid appearance is addressed without restoring midface support. By correcting the structural framework that supports the eyelid, the DeepFrame Facelift™ provides a stable and natural foundation for periorbital rejuvenation while avoiding the distortions commonly associated with superficial intervention.

CHAPTER 5

How the DeepFrame Facelift™ Addresses the Midface

The midface occupies a central position in both the anatomy of the face and the process of facial aging. Its contours shape the appearance of the eyes, define the prominence and curvature of the cheeks, influence the depth and character of the nasolabial fold, and exert a profound effect on the mechanical load borne by the lower face and neck. Despite this central role, the midface has historically been one of the most inconsistently and inadequately treated regions in facelift surgery. This inconsistency arises not from lack of importance, but from the fact that midface aging occurs primarily at a deeper anatomical level than many traditional techniques are designed to address.

The DeepFrame Facelift™ places midface correction at the core of its structural philosophy. Rather than attempting to influence midface appearance indirectly through lateral traction or superficial tightening, it restores midface position at the level where aging originates. This approach reflects a recognition that meaningful rejuvenation of the midface requires restoration of anatomy rather than manipulation of surface contour.

To understand why midface correction is so critical, it is necessary to examine the structural mechanisms that drive aging in this region. Midface aging is not a superficial phenomenon. It is the result of a convergence of skeletal remodeling, ligamentous attenuation, and displacement of deep fat compartments, all of which interact to alter the spatial relationships that once produced youthful contour.[1-4,10,11]

With advancing age, the maxilla undergoes gradual retrusion. This change reduces anterior projection beneath the orbit and diminishes the bony platform that supports the cheek.[4] At the same time, resorption of the infraorbital rim further weakens structural support in the periorbital region. These skeletal changes alone do not dramatically alter appearance, but they create a permissive environment for soft tissue descent.

Retaining ligaments that once stabilized the midface elongate over time. Rather than rupturing, they gradually lose tensile strength, allowing increased mobility of the cheek relative to fixed skeletal landmarks. Deep fat compartments, particularly the deep medial cheek fat and the suborbicularis oculi fat, respond to this loss of support by migrating inferiorly. Importantly, this migration reflects displacement rather than true loss of tissue.[1,2] In most patients, deep fat volume remains present but is no longer located where it once contributed to youthful contour.

The visible consequences of these changes follow a characteristic pattern. The malar eminence flattens as deep fat descends away from its youthful position. The cheek migrates inferiorly and posteriorly, increasing the distance between the lower eyelid and the cheek. Fixed anatomical boundaries such as the nasolabial fold become more prominent as mobile tissues descend against regions of relative fixation. The face appears longer, heavier, and less structurally supported, even in the absence of significant skin laxity.

When these structural changes are not corrected, attempts to rejuvenate the midface remain incomplete regardless of surface improvement. Skin tightening may temporarily smooth contours, and volumetric treatments may soften hollows, but neither approach restores the underlying anatomy that governs midface form and stability. As a result, such interventions often produce transient or artificial results.

The defining midface maneuver of the DeepFrame Facelift™ is elevation in the subperiosteal deep plane. This approach reflects an understanding that midface aging originates at the interface between soft tissue and bone. By releasing the midface at its skeletal attachment, tissues can be mobilized as a cohesive unit and repositioned superiorly and anteriorly in a stable and anatomically coherent manner.[10,11]

Subperiosteal elevation directly restores the relationship between the cheek, the orbit, and the maxilla. Because correction occurs at the depth where aging originates, it does not depend on skin tension or superficial fixation. Instead, repositioned tissues are supported at the periosteal level, which provides a durable and mechanically sound foundation. This distinction is critical for both the natural appearance and longevity of the result.

By contrast, attempts to elevate the midface through superficial or lateral traction often fail to restore true position. Lateral pull redistributes tissue without addressing vertical descent. It may create the illusion of improvement in certain views while flattening malar projection and distorting facial curvature. Subperiosteal elevation avoids these pitfalls by restoring tissues along their original vector of descent and anchoring them at their anatomical origin.

Restoration of malar projection is one of the most visually significant outcomes of structural midface correction. Youthful midface aesthetics are characterized by smooth convexity over the malar eminence and gentle transitions between facial units. This curvature reflects the natural relationship between the cheek fat compartments and the underlying skeleton. As the midface

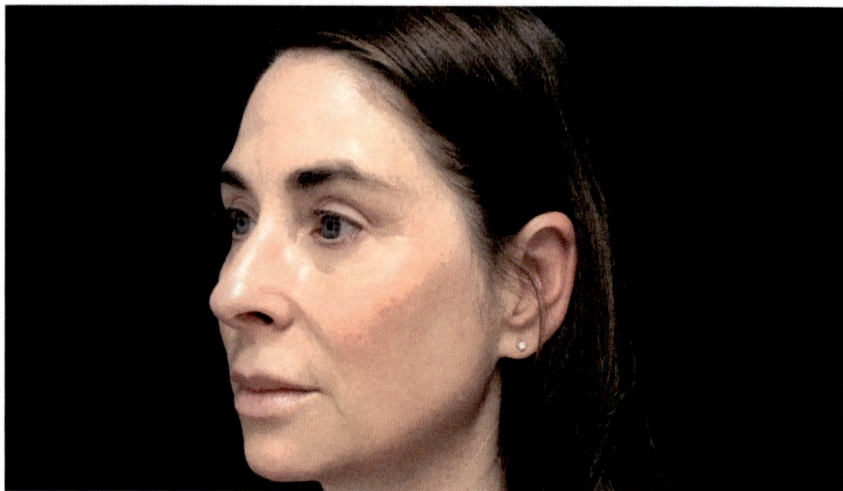

Following deep plane midface elevation during
DeepFrame Facelift™, the malar cheek projection is
improved, and the lower lid is shortened.

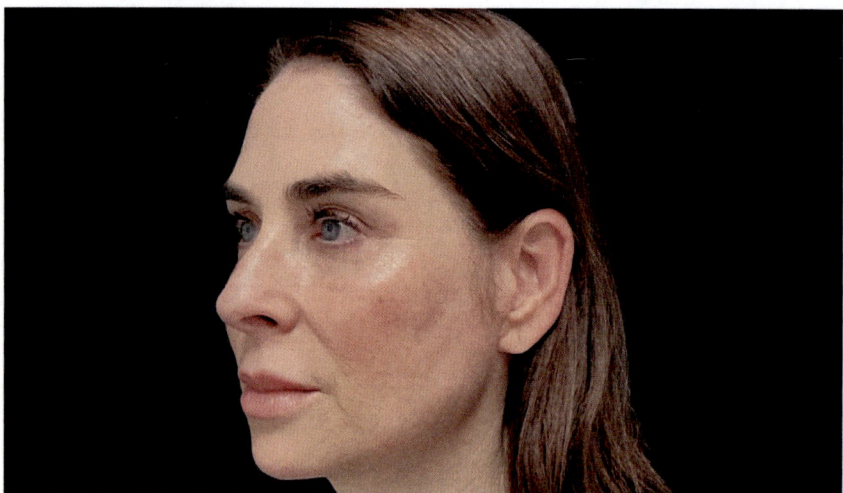

descends, these transitions become abrupt, and the face appears flattened or heavy.

The DeepFrame Facelift™ restores malar projection by repositioning native tissues rather than adding volume. This distinction is essential. Volumetric augmentation can increase fullness, but it does not recreate the spatial relationships that define youthful contour. In some cases, it exaggerates heaviness or produces an augmented appearance that conflicts with the patient's skeletal anatomy.

By contrast, repositioning existing tissues in the deep plane restores prominence in a manner consistent with the individual's bone structure. The cheek regains its natural curvature without appearing artificial or overfilled. Because correction respects native anatomy, results remain individualized rather than conforming to a standardized aesthetic ideal. This preservation of individuality is a hallmark of structural rejuvenation.

Midfacial elevation and stabilization are performed through the eyelid incisions during a DeepFrame Facelift™. This minimally invasive technique powerfully provides access to the cheek tissue at the malar region, and suspension of the deep plane tissue to the temporalis fascia and lateral orbit allows for long-lasting stability. While this approach serves to improve lower lid aesthetics and support the lower lid tissue, the resuspension of tissue addresses shadows of aging like no other maneuver. The shadow of the lateral cheek descent is removed, and the nasolabial crease is rejuvenated as the overlying tissue is newly supported.

The influence of midface position on the nasolabial fold provides another example of why structural correction is superior to surface manipulation. The nasolabial fold is frequently targeted directly with fillers, yet its prominence is largely a consequence of midface descent. It represents a boundary between relatively fixed tissues anchored to the maxilla and more mobile tissues above.

When the midface descends, mobile tissues accumulate against this fixed boundary, deepening the fold. Directly filling the fold does not address the cause of this accumulation. While such approaches may soften the fold temporarily, they often compromise natural movement or create stiffness. Repeated injections of the fold create abnormal contours that are easily evident to even the untrained eye.

The DeepFrame Facelift™ improves the nasolabial fold indirectly by restoring the position of tissues above it. As the cheek is elevated subperiosteally, tension across the fold decreases, and its depth softens naturally. This approach preserves animation and avoids the unnatural appearance that can result from aggressive direct treatment. The fold is not eliminated, but it becomes consistent with a youthful facial structure.

Midface descent also plays a critical role in accelerating the aging of the lower face and neck. As the cheek migrates inferiorly, it increases mechanical load on the superficial musculoaponeurotic system and the platysma. This added load contributes to jowl formation, loss of jawline definition, and cervical laxity. In this way, midface aging acts as a driver of changes that extend well beyond its own anatomical boundaries. [3,8,14]

By restoring midface position, the DeepFrame Facelift™ reduces inferior vector forces transmitted to the lower face. This offloading enhances the effectiveness and longevity of lower face and neck correction. Procedures performed below the midface are not forced to compensate for ongoing downward pressure from above. Instead, they function within a rebalanced mechanical environment.

This concept underscores the role of the midface as a structural linchpin in facial aging. Correction at this level stabilizes the entire cervicofacial complex. Conversely, failure to address midface descent undermines even technically precise lower face or neck procedures. The DeepFrame approach recognizes this interdependence and places midface restoration at the center of comprehensive

Figure 4

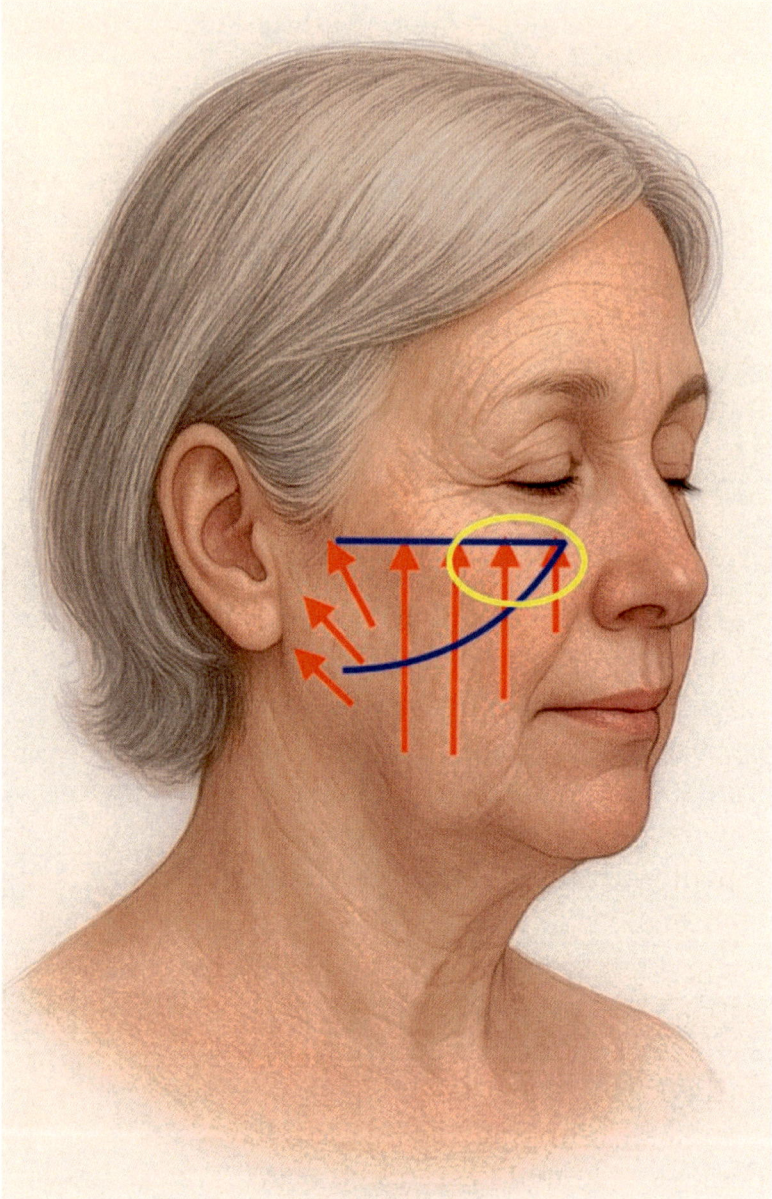

Increasing magnitude of vertical vectors laterally
creates redundancy at the cheek apex adding volume
without filler or fat graft (yellow circle)

rejuvenation.

Integration with adjacent regions is therefore a defining feature of midface correction in the DeepFrame Facelift™. Elevation of the cheek improves periorbital contour by restoring support beneath the lower eyelid. It reduces strain on the lower face by decreasing the inferior load. It influences global facial balance by reestablishing appropriate proportions between the upper, middle, and lower thirds of the face.

This integrated approach contrasts with techniques that treat facial regions in isolation. Fragmented correction may produce localized improvement but often results in disharmony. Youthful eyes above a descended midface or a tightened neck beneath an unsupported jawline appear incongruent. Structural midface correction helps prevent such discordance by restoring the anatomical relationships that unify the face.

Another advantage of subperiosteal deep plane midface elevation is its effect on durability. Because tissues are repositioned and supported at the level of periosteum, they are less susceptible to stretching or relapse. Fixation is inherently more stable than superficial anchoring, and the mechanical forces acting on repositioned tissues are reduced rather than merely resisted. As a result, midface correction achieved through the

DeepFrame Facelift™ ages more gracefully over time.

Importantly, this approach does not seek to freeze the face or eliminate all signs of aging. Instead, it establishes a new anatomical baseline from which aging resumes in a more favorable configuration. The midface remains supported, contours remain harmonious, and changes occur gradually rather than abruptly.

The midface has long been a source of controversy in facelift surgery precisely because it demands deeper anatomical engagement. Techniques that avoid this depth may appear safer or simpler, but they sacrifice the opportunity for true structural correction. The experienced surgeon recognizes the safety of this deep plane, and the DeepFrame Facelift™ embraces this complexity, recognizing that meaningful rejuvenation requires addressing the root causes of aging rather than its surface manifestations.

In summary, the midface is a structural linchpin of facial aging. Its descent alters facial contour, disrupts periorbital support, deepens fixed folds, and increases mechanical load on the lower face and neck. The DeepFrame Facelift™ addresses midface aging through true subperiosteal elevation, restoring anatomical relationships rather than camouflaging their disruption.

By correcting the midface at its anatomical origin, the DeepFrame approach produces natural contour, stabilizes adjacent regions, and establishes a foundation for durable facial rejuvenation. This structural restoration not only improves midface aesthetics but also enhances the effectiveness and longevity of correction throughout the face and neck, reinforcing the central role of the midface in comprehensive rejuvenation.

CHAPTER 5A

Common Errors When the Midface Is Treated Superficially

Errors in midface rejuvenation most often arise from underestimating the depth at which midface aging occurs. Because changes in this region can sometimes be softened temporarily through surface manipulation, superficial approaches remain common despite their inability to correct the underlying structural problem. While these methods may produce short-term visual improvement, they frequently lead to distortion, imbalance, or early relapse as deeper forces continue to act unopposed.

One of the most persistent errors is reliance on lateral or posterolateral traction to influence the midface. Lateral pulling may smooth skin and reduce the appearance of folds transiently, but it does not restore vertical cheek position or malar projection. Because the dominant vector of midface aging is vertical descent, lateral correction is biomechanically inefficient. Over time, it tends to flatten the cheek, widen the face, and redirect tissues along unnatural paths. As a result, any apparent improvement is unstable and prone to recurrence.

78

Another common error is treating midface descent as though it were primarily a problem of volume loss. Flattening of the cheek and hollowing beneath the eye are often interpreted as deficiencies rather than as consequences of displacement. This assumption leads to filler placement or fat grafting into a descended structure without restoring its position. Adding volume to a structure that has migrated inferiorly increases mass without improving support. Over time, this can worsen heaviness, blur anatomical landmarks, and accelerate further descent. Repeated volumization frequently produces an overfilled appearance that obscures natural facial architecture.

Direct treatment of the nasolabial fold represents a related superficial strategy. Because the fold is visually prominent, it is often targeted directly with fillers or surgical manipulation. However, the nasolabial fold exists largely because tissues above it have descended against a fixed boundary.[1,5] Treating the fold without elevating the midface addresses the symptom rather than the cause. This approach may stiffen facial movement, create unnatural transitions between facial units, and fail to provide durable improvement.

Superficial midface treatments also commonly ignore the contribution of skeletal remodeling. Retraction of the maxilla and loss of infraorbital projection alter the foundation upon which midface soft tissues rest. Without acknowledging this changing support, attempts to improve surface contour remain incomplete. Soft tissues cannot be meaningfully repositioned if their skeletal reference point is not considered.

Fragmented regional planning further undermines midface outcomes. The midface influences the appearance of the eyes and the mechanical load borne by the lower face and neck. Treating it independently often produces discordant results, such as periorbital improvement above an unsupported cheek or lower face tightening beneath a descended midface. These imbalances reflect conceptual rather than technical failure.[26,27]

Superficial treatment of midface aging may offer transient improvement, but it does so without correcting the displacement that drives visible change. Errors arise when lateral traction substitutes for vertical repositioning, when volume is added instead of restoring structure, and when regional planning is fragmented. By addressing the midface at the level of skeletal attachment and integrating correction across facial regions, the DeepFrame Facelift™ avoids these pitfalls and restores the midface as a stabilizing center of facial architecture.

CHAPTER 6

How the DeepFrame Facelift™ Addresses the Lower Face

The lower face is one of the most visually defining regions of facial aging. Changes in this area are readily perceived and strongly influence judgments of age, health, and vitality. Loss of jawline definition, formation of jowls, and disruption of the smooth transition between cheek and mandible are among the most recognizable manifestations of facial aging. Although these features are often attributed to skin laxity, such an explanation is incomplete. In reality, the visible changes of the lower face are the surface expression of deeper structural failure involving the superficial musculoaponeurotic system, the distribution of mechanical load across facial regions, and the continuity of support between the face and neck. [5,8,14]

The DeepFrame Facelift™ addresses the lower face through anatomically guided restoration of deep support rather than through superficial tightening. This approach recognizes that the lower face is not a passive region of skin redundancy, but a dynamic anatomical zone that must balance structural correction with preservation of movement, expression, and identity. Effective rejuvenation of the lower face therefore depends on restoring the mechanical environment in which soft tissues function, rather than imposing tension at the surface.

Lower face aging reflects progressive elongation and weakening of the superficial musculoaponeurotic system (SMAS), compounded by increasing inferior load transmitted from the descending midface.[5,9,14] In youth, the SMAS functions as a load-bearing fascial network that suspends the soft tissues of the face over the mandibular border. Its integrity allows the jawline to remain defined and the transition between cheek and mandible to appear smooth and continuous.

With age, the SMAS gradually elongates and loses tensile integrity. This change does not occur uniformly across the face. In the lower face, elongation of the SMAS is particularly consequential because it allows soft tissues that were once supported above the mandibular border to migrate downward and inward. At the same time, descent of the midface increases inferior vector forces acting on the lower face, accelerating the failure of SMAS support.

The resulting tissue migration produces a characteristic pattern of aging. Soft tissues accumulate along the mandibular border, forming jowls.[5,6,9] The pre-jowl sulcus deepens as tissue descends away from the parasymphyseal region. The mandibular border loses definition as mobile tissues encroach upon a region that was once sharply contoured. Skin follows the position of deeper tissues and therefore mirrors, rather than causes, these changes. Attribution of jowl formation primarily to skin laxity misunderstands the sequence of events that produce lower face aging.

Addressing skin laxity alone cannot restore jawline contour if deep support remains compromised. Skin tightening may temporarily sharpen the mandibular border, but it does so by placing tension on tissues not designed to bear sustained load. Over time, this tension leads to stretching, distortion, and recurrence of laxity as deeper structures continue to fail.

A central principle of the DeepFrame Facelift™ is recognition that the SMAS is a continuous structure with regional variability. Although it spans the face and neck, its thickness, strength, and contribution to aging differ between the midface, lower face, and cervical region. As a result, uniform manipulation of the SMAS fails to address the specific mechanical failures that occur in each area.

In the lower face, the DeepFrame approach employs region-specific SMAS manipulation tailored to the patient's tissue quality, degree of descent, and overall facial architecture. In patients with heavier soft tissue or advanced jowl formation, sub-SMAS mobilization and potential SMASectomy at the deep plane allows elevation of the soft-tissue envelope as a cohesive unit. This maneuver restores the position of tissues relative to the mandible without relying on skin tension. The removal of SMAS tissue in the full face aids in sculpting the natural curvature of youth while limiting facial widening.

In patients with milder descent or thinner facial structure, deep plane SMAS plication or reinforcement may be required to restore fascial support without extensive release. Plication of SMAS tissue in the thinner face allows for volumetric augmentation of the cheek without the addition of fillers.

The goal of SMAS manipulation in the DeepFrame Facelift™ is not maximal tightening, but restoration of normal tension and position relative to the zygoma and mandibular border. Excessive tightening risks distortion of facial movement and produces an operated appearance. Insufficient support fails to correct contour. The balance lies in restoring the SMAS to a state in which it can once again function as a stable suspensory structure.

Vector planning plays a decisive role in lower face correction. The lower face does not age along a single axis. Jowl formation reflects both vertical descent and inferomedial migration of soft tissues as SMAS support weakens. Effective correction therefore requires composite vectors that elevate tissues superiorly while refining contour laterally.

The DeepFrame Facelift™ applies vertical support medially to lift jowl tissue back into the cheek, restoring continuity between the midface and lower face. This medial vertical component addresses the true direction of descent and reduces the volume of tissue accumulating along the jawline. At the same time, oblique refinement laterally restores mandibular definition without widening the face or distorting the oral commissure.

Importantly, more elevation of lateral SMAS is possible as compared to the medial SMAS, as the mobility of the jowl and neck tissue allows greater upward motion in this area. The differential in degree of lift from medial to lateral creates an angle of deep plane elevation based on the magnitude of the vectors in addition to their direction. As the lateral elevation is in excess of the medial elevation, a redundancy or "dog ear" of deep plane tissue develops at the apex of the medial cheek, providing ideal volume in this area.(Figure 4) This natural volume once again precludes the need for fat grafting or filler to maximize the ideal "Ogee Curve" that reflects the youthful facial contour.

The balanced vector strategy contrasts with approaches that rely primarily on lateral pull.

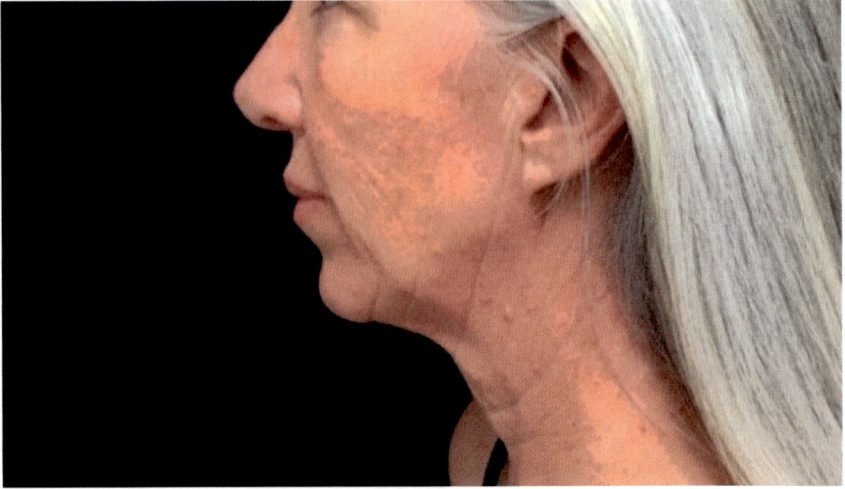

Deep plane midface elevation while addressing the SMAS in the lower face improves lower face redundancy and associated shadows while defining the mandibular border and improving the neck contour.

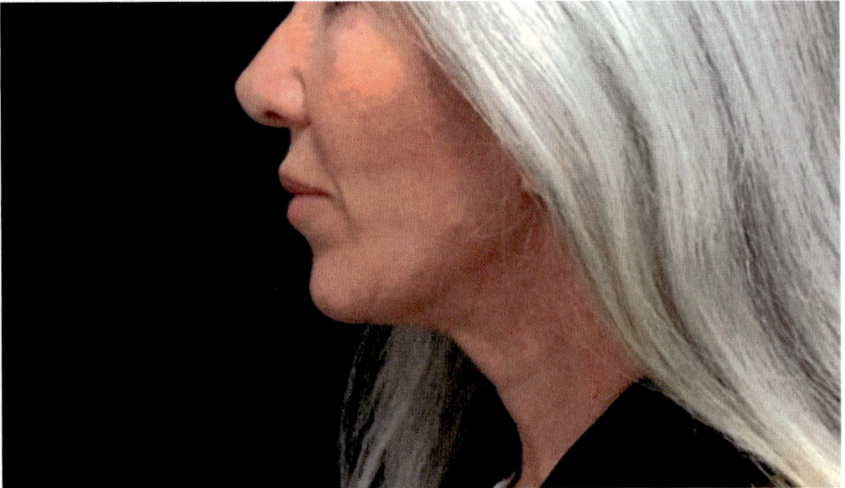

Excessive lateral traction may sharpen the jawline temporarily, but it often widens the face, displaces tissues unnaturally, and places stress on fixation points. Over time, these forces contribute to relapse and distortion. By aligning correction with anatomical vectors, the DeepFrame approach restores jawline contour without producing rigidity or an over-tightened appearance.

Integration with the midface is essential for durable lower face correction. Descent of the midface increases inferior load on the SMAS and accelerates jowl formation. Treating the lower face in isolation may produce short-term improvement, but uncorrected midface descent continues to exert downward pressure, undermining the result.

The DeepFrame Facelift™ integrates lower face correction with subperiosteal midface elevation. By restoring midface position, inferior forces acting on the lower face are reduced at their source. This offloading effect enhances the effectiveness and longevity of jawline correction. Lower face tissues are no longer required to compensate for ongoing descent above them. Instead, they function within a rebalanced mechanical environment.

This integration reinforces the concept that facial regions do not age independently. The lower face serves as a transitional zone between the midface and neck. Its appearance reflects the balance of forces acting from above and below. Addressing only one component of this system produces incomplete and unstable results.[5][8]

Integration with the neck further strengthens lower face outcomes. The lower face and neck function as a continuous unit through the SMAS platysma complex. Loss of mandibular definition is closely linked to platysmal elongation, medial separation, and cervical descent.[21,22] Treating the lower face without addressing the neck often leaves the jawline unsupported inferiorly, resulting in blunting of contour or early recurrence of laxity.

The DeepFrame Facelift™ coordinates lower face SMAS support with cervical vector planning. By restoring continuity of the cervicofacial sling, jawline definition is reinforced from below as well as above. This integration produces a smoother transition between face and neck and contributes to a more stable cervicomental angle. The result is not only aesthetic improvement, but structural coherence.

Preservation of expression and function is a critical consideration in lower face rejuvenation. The lower face plays a central role in speech, mastication, and emotional expression. Overcorrection can result in stiffness, asymmetry, or distortion of the oral commissure. These outcomes are particularly distressing because they alter the patient's expressive identity.

By placing corrective forces in deep layers rather than skin, and by respecting regional vector requirements, the DeepFrame Facelift™ preserves natural movement while restoring contour. Muscles operate within restored anatomical boundaries rather than against imposed tension. Skin redrapes passively over a supported framework rather than serving as a load-bearing structure. As a result, expression is maintained even as contour is improved.

Another advantage of deep plane structural correction is its effect on longevity. Corrections achieved through deep support require less sustained tension and place less stress on fixation points. As a result, they age more gracefully and predictably. The lower face does not remain frozen in a youthful configuration, but it retains structural coherence as aging resumes from a corrected baseline.

The DeepFrame approach does not seek to eliminate all signs of aging in the lower face. Instead, it aims to restore anatomical relationships that allow aging to proceed in a balanced and harmonious manner. This perspective aligns surgical planning with biological reality and shapes patient expectations toward durability rather than permanence.

In summary, lower face aging is fundamentally a structural problem driven by elongation of the

SMAS, displacement of soft tissues, and increasing inferior load transmitted from the midface. The DeepFrame Facelift™ addresses these changes through region-specific deep plane SMAS manipulation, precise vector control, and integration with midface and neck correction.

By restoring deep plane support rather than tightening skin, the DeepFrame approach produces natural jawline definition, preserves expression, augments the cheek naturally, and contributes to durable facial rejuvenation. The lower face is restored not as an isolated aesthetic unit, but as an integral component of a unified cervicofacial framework.

CHAPTER 6A

Common Errors When the Lower Face Is Treated Superficially

Errors in lower face rejuvenation most often stem from misunderstanding the structural nature of jowl formation and jawline deterioration. Because these changes are visually prominent, superficial treatments remain attractive and widely used. While such approaches may produce immediate surface improvement, they fail to correct the deeper anatomical failures that drive lower face aging. Over time, this disconnect leads to distortion, early relapse, and results that appear increasingly unnatural.

One of the most frequent errors is treating jowls as a problem of excess skin. Skin excision or lateral tightening can temporarily smooth the surface of the lower face, but it does not reposition the descended superficial musculoaponeurotic system or reduce the inferior load transmitted from the midface. As a result, the apparent improvement is unstable. Jowls often recur as deeper tissues continue to migrate, sometimes in a more distorted configuration as skin tension redistributes forces unpredictably. This creates the classic "swept" look, where lateral tension lines are evident in the facial skin and are a classic inicator of having had "work done."

Uniform lateral pulling represents another common superficial strategy. Lateral traction may tighten the jawline transiently, but it does not address the vertical and inferomedial vectors along which lower face aging occurs. By redirecting tissues laterally rather than restoring them superiorly, this approach risks widening the lower face, flattening natural curvature, and altering the shape or position of the oral commissure. Over time, these changes contribute to a pulled appearance that conflicts with natural facial proportions.

Excessive reliance on skin tension further undermines lower face outcomes. Skin is not designed to function as a primary load-bearing structure. When it is used to support deeper tissues, it predictably stretches, scars widen, and contour deteriorates. Increased tension also raises the risk of delayed healing and visible scarring. Superficial tightening may therefore appear effective in the short term while actively compromising long-term stability and aesthetics.

The use of fillers to camouflage jowls or pre jowl hollowing reflects a similar misunderstanding of cause and effect. Injecting volume into these regions may temporarily smooth contour irregularities, but it does not restore SMAS position or reduce mechanical load. Added volume can blur mandibular definition and increase heaviness in a region where sharp contour is desirable. Repeated filler treatments often complicate future surgical correction by obscuring tissue planes and altering anatomy.

Failure to coordinate lower face correction with midface and neck support represents a more global planning error. The lower face exists within a continuous cervicofacial system. Descent of the midface increases inferior load, and platysmal weakening undermines mandibular definition from below. Treating the jawline without addressing these adjacent regions often produces imbalance and early recurrence of laxity. Superficial approaches frequently fragment facial planning by focusing on visible features rather than structural relationships.[26,27]

Superficial treatment of lower face aging prioritizes short term appearance over anatomical correction. Errors arise when jowls are treated as skin problems, when lateral traction substitutes for vertical support, and when integration with the midface and neck is ignored.[5,9,22] By restoring SMAS integrity, aligning vectors with true aging patterns, and coordinating correction across facial regions, the DeepFrame Facelift™ avoids these pitfalls and provides a stable and natural foundation for lower face rejuvenation.

CHAPTER 7

How the DeepFrame Facelift™ Addresses the Neck

The neck occupies a uniquely revealing position in facial aging. Changes in cervical contour are among the most immediately recognizable signs of age and are often cited by patients as a source of dissatisfaction even when other facial regions appear relatively preserved. Loss of cervical definition, blunting of the cervicomental angle, platysmal banding, and submental fullness all contribute to an aged appearance that is difficult to conceal. Despite this visibility, the neck has frequently been treated as an isolated aesthetic unit, addressed independently from the face through skin tightening or limited platysmal manipulation. Such approaches underestimate the degree to which cervical aging reflects failure of a broader cervicofacial support system rather than a localized neck problem.[18-20]

The DeepFrame Facelift™ approaches the neck as an integral structural extension of the face. Cervical correction is planned and executed in continuity with midface and lower face restoration. This strategy recognizes that durable neck rejuvenation depends on restoring the mechanical integrity of the superficial musculoaponeurotic system and platysma as a unified structure, reestablishing appropriate vector support, and reducing inferior load transmitted from the aging face above. By addressing these factors collectively, the DeepFrame approach restores cervical contour in a manner that is both natural in appearance and stable over time.

In youth, the neck is supported by a coordinated system of anatomical structures that function together to maintain contour and definition. The platysma forms a broad, thin muscular sheet that extends from the lower face into the neck, contributing to mandibular definition and the cervicomental angle. This muscle is reinforced by the deep cervical fascia and functions in continuity with the inferior extension of the superficial musculo-aponeurotic system. Together, these elements create a cervicofacial sling that suspends soft tissues, distributes mechanical load, and allows dynamic movement without loss of contour. [19,20,24]

When this system is intact, the mandibular border appears crisp, the cervicomental angle is well defined, and the transition between face and neck is smooth and harmonious. The neck does not function as an isolated column of skin and fat, but as the inferior expression of facial structure. This integrated anatomy explains why youthful neck appearance depends as much on facial support as on cervical tissue quality.

With aging, this coordinated support system progressively weakens. The platysma elongates and loses tone. Medial separation of the platysmal edges becomes apparent, leading to banding during animation and, eventually, at rest. The inferior extension of the SMAS loses tensile strength, reducing its ability to suspend cervical soft tissues. At the same time, descent of the midface and lower face increases inferior vector forces transmitted into the neck. Subcutaneous tissues descend and accumulate, and the cervicomental angle becomes obtuse as deep support fails.

These changes rarely occur in isolation. Cervical aging is almost always compounded by uncorrected descent of the face above. When midface and lower face support deteriorate, the neck becomes the repository for inferior load. Treating the neck without addressing these upstream forces is therefore inherently unstable. Even technically precise cervical procedures are undermined if the face continues to descend and transmit strain into the neck.

A central principle of the DeepFrame Facelift™ is recognition of the SMAS and platysma as a continuous anatomical structure rather than separate entities. Historically, facial and neck procedures have often been compartmentalized, with distinct operations applied to each region. This fragmentation disrupts anatomical continuity and limits durability. When the neck is tightened independently of the face, tension is concentrated at artificial boundaries, increasing the risk of recurrence and distortion.

The DeepFrame approach restores cervicofacial continuity by coordinating lower face SMAS manipulation with platysmal support. When the SMAS is repositioned and reinforced superiorly, strain on the platysma is reduced. Cervical correction can then be achieved with less force and greater mechanical efficiency. Rather than forcing the neck into position, the procedure reestablishes the conditions under which the neck can maintain its contour naturally.

Vector planning plays a critical role in cervical rejuvenation. Cervical aging follows predictable inferior and anterior vectors as the platysma elongates and deep support weakens. Effective correction must counter these forces without introducing unnatural tension or contour distortion. Superficial tightening often attempts to pull the neck skin posteriorly, but this does not address the vertical component of descent and may create irregularities or a bound-down appearance.

The DeepFrame Facelift™ applies vertical and superolateral support through deep structures rather than relying on skin tension. Platysmal correction is performed in a manner that restores its function as a dynamic support structure. By repositioning and reinforcing the platysma within the context of a restored SMAS, the neck regains its ability to maintain contour during both rest and movement. This approach avoids the stiff or artificial appearance that can result from excessive superficial tightening.

Management of platysmal banding illustrates the importance of structural thinking in cervical rejuvenation. Platysmal bands are often treated as isolated muscular defects, addressed through direct excision or aggressive tightening. While such interventions may temporarily reduce the appearance of bands, they do not address the underlying failure of the cervicofacial sling. Without restoring global support, banding often recurs or is replaced by other contour irregularities.

Restoration of the cervicomental angle depends on deep support rather than skin manipulation. A sharp cervicomental angle is a hallmark of youthful neck anatomy, but attempts to recreate it through skin excision or aggressive tightening often produce unnatural transitions or visible scarring. In contrast, when deep structures are repositioned and supported, the cervicomental angle sharpens as a natural consequence of restored anatomy. The angle is not forced into position but reemerges as the cervicofacial framework is reestablished.

When required, a platysmaplasty with back-cutting of the platysmal bands can be a powerful tool in the DeepFrame procedure. This maneuver, however, is not always required nor beneficial. The cervicofacial structure of the individual is always evaluated, discussed, and addressed accordingly for each patient. An acute cervicomental angle in a round face, for example, will appear mismatched and inappropriate.

Similarly, excessive fat resection or liposuction must be avoided in order to prevent submental skeletalization or hollowing of this region. An operated appearance of the neck can be an unwelcome sequelae of poor planning, and the deep tissues and fat of the neck must be managed appropriately

Integration with facial correction is essential for durable neck rejuvenation. Midface elevation reduces the downward pull on the lower face. Lower face support stabilizes the mandibular border. When these corrections are performed in concert with cervical restoration, the neck benefits from a reduction in mechanical stress. The result is not only improved contour but also enhanced longevity.

The DeepFrame Facelift™ therefore treats the neck as the inferior expression of facial structure rather than as a separate aesthetic unit. This perspective shifts the focus from surface appearance to underlying mechanics. Cervical rejuvenation becomes a process of restoring balance within a continuous anatomical system rather than imposing isolated corrections.

Preservation of natural movement is another critical consideration in neck rejuvenation. The neck is highly dynamic, participating in speech, swallowing, and head movement. Over tightening or excessive superficial correction can restrict motion, produce discomfort, or create an unnatural appearance that is particularly noticeable during animation. Patients may perceive such outcomes as stiffness or tightness even when static contour appears improved.

By placing corrective forces in deep layers and minimizing reliance on skin tension, the DeepFrame approach preserves natural cervical movement. Muscles and soft tissues operate within restored anatomical boundaries rather than against imposed constraints. Skin redrapes passively over a supported framework, allowing motion without distortion. This preservation of function contributes significantly to patient satisfaction and long term acceptance of the result.

Longevity of cervical rejuvenation is closely linked to biomechanical efficiency. Corrections that require sustained tension are inherently vulnerable to relapse as tissues stretch and fixation points fatigue. In contrast, corrections that restore anatomical relationships reduce the forces acting on tissues and allow them to age more gracefully. The DeepFrame approach emphasizes this principle by restoring deep support and reducing inferior load rather than resisting it.

Importantly, the DeepFrame Facelift™ does not seek to eliminate all signs of aging in the neck. Aging is a continuous biological process that cannot be halted surgically. Instead, the procedure establishes a new anatomical baseline by correcting accumulated structural distortions. From this point, aging resumes in a more favorable configuration, with preserved contour and harmony.

This perspective shapes both surgical planning and patient counseling. Expectations are framed around durability and natural progression rather than permanence. Patients understand that the goal is restoration of structure rather than indefinite prevention of change. This alignment between surgical intent and biological reality contributes to long term satisfaction.

In summary, cervical aging reflects failure of a continuous cervicofacial support system rather than isolated neck laxity. Loss of platysmal integrity, elongation of the SMAS, and increased inferior load from the aging face interact to produce visible cervical changes. Superficial treatments that focus on skin tightening or isolated band correction fail to address these underlying mechanisms.

The DeepFrame Facelift™ addresses the neck by restoring SMAS platysma continuity, aligning vectors with true aging patterns, and integrating cervical correction with midface and lower face support. By reestablishing deep structural balance, the approach produces a defined, natural appearing neck that harmonizes with facial rejuvenation and maintains its result over time.

CHAPTER 7A

Common Errors When the Neck Is Treated Superficially

The neck is one of the most frequently misunderstood regions in facial rejuvenation. Its visible changes are often attributed to skin laxity or fat accumulation, leading to treatments that focus on surface tightening or isolated contouring maneuvers. While such approaches may produce short-term improvement, they fail to address the structural relationships that govern cervical form and stability. Over time, these errors commonly result in recurrence, distortion, or disharmony between the face and neck.

A primary error in superficial neck treatment is the assumption that cervical aging is an isolated phenomenon. In reality, the neck is the inferior extension of the facial support system. Loss of mandibular definition, platysmal banding, and blunting of the cervicomental angle frequently reflect failure of the SMAS platysma complex combined with inferior load transmitted from the descending midface and lower face. Treating the neck without addressing these upstream contributors places corrective forces at a mechanical disadvantage and undermines durability.

Another common error is reliance on skin tightening as the principal method of correction. Skin in the neck is thin, highly mobile, and poorly suited to bear sustained tension. When tightened without restoration of deep support, it stretches predictably over time. This not only leads to early recurrence of laxity, but also increases the risk of widened scars, contour irregularities, and an operated appearance. Skin tightening may temporarily improve surface smoothness, but it does not restore cervical architecture.

Superficial treatment often focuses narrowly on platysmal bands as discrete problems rather than as manifestations of broader structural failure. Isolated band excision or plication may flatten visible cords in the short term, but without restoring platysmal tension within a continuous cervicofacial framework, bands frequently recur or reappear asymmetrically. The platysma functions as part of a sling, not as an independent structure, and its behavior cannot be normalized without addressing its superior attachments and load environment.

Another frequent error is aggressive submental fat removal without restoring structural support. While excess submental fat can contribute to cervical fullness, over-resection in the absence of deep support exaggerates skin laxity and may produce an aged or skeletonized appearance. Removal of volume without repositioning the platysma or reinforcing mandibular support often worsens long-term contour. The subcutaneous fat of the cervicomental region contributes to the smoothing of the contour of the neck, and over-resection of the fat in this region is often mistakenly performed as a "minimally invasive" option. Skeletalization of the submental musculature is an unnatural sign of poor surgical decision making, as is hollowing under the chin from over-resection during liposuction.

Fragmented regional planning also undermines cervical outcomes. Treating the neck independently from the lower face can create visible discontinuities at the mandibular border. A tightened neck beneath an unsupported jawline appears artificial and unstable. Conversely, lower face correction without cervical integration leaves inferior laxity unaddressed. Harmonious rejuvenation requires coordinated correction across regions.

Superficial approaches may also underestimate the importance of vector planning. Cervical aging follows inferior and anterior vectors. Lateral tightening alone does not counter these forces effectively and may distort natural contours. When vectors are misaligned, results deteriorate rapidly despite initial improvement.

Finally, superficial treatment strategies often prioritize immediacy over longevity. Short recovery and minimal invasiveness are appealing, but when structural failure is present, such approaches merely delay definitive correction. Repeated superficial interventions can complicate future surgery by altering tissue planes and vascularity.

In contrast, structural correction of the neck maximizes continuity of the SMAS platysma complex, redistributes load, and allows skin to redrape without tension. By addressing cervical aging as part of an integrated facial system, durable contour and natural appearance can be achieved.

CHAPTER 8

The Advantages of the DeepFrame Facelift™ Over Filler and Fat Grafting

Over the past two decades, injectable fillers and fat grafting have become central tools in facial rejuvenation. Their widespread adoption reflects both technological advances and shifting patient preferences toward minimally invasive interventions. These modalities offer convenience, relatively short recovery periods, and the perception of reversibility. In selected circumstances, they can provide meaningful aesthetic benefit. However, their limitations become increasingly evident when they are used as primary strategies to address facial aging driven by structural descent rather than true volume deficiency.

The DeepFrame Facelift™ offers a fundamentally different solution. Instead of compensating for displacement with added material, it restores native tissues to their anatomically appropriate positions. This distinction is not merely technical. It represents a different understanding of how faces age and how rejuvenation should be achieved. The implications of this difference extend to facial harmony, longevity of results, preservation of expression, and long term tissue health.

To appreciate the advantages of structural repositioning over volumetric augmentation, it is necessary to examine the assumptions that underlie filler and fat grafting strategies and to contrast them with the anatomical realities of facial aging.

A central misconception in modern facial rejuvenation is the assumption that aging primarily reflects volume loss. This view is reinforced by the visible appearance of hollows, flattening, and contour changes that seem to suggest deflation. While selective volume loss does occur, particularly in superficial fat compartments and in certain skeletal regions, the dominant process in midface and lower face aging is displacement of deep tissues rather than global deficiency.

As skeletal support diminishes and retaining ligaments attenuate, deep fat compartments migrate inferiorly and medially. The cheek descends away from the orbit. Soft tissues accumulate against fixed anatomical boundaries such as the nasolabial fold and mandibular border. These shifts alter contour and create the visual impression of hollowing in some areas and fullness in others, even though total tissue volume may be relatively preserved.

When displaced structures are treated as if they were deficient, volume is added to a malpositioned framework. This increases mass without restoring architecture. The underlying relationships among bone, fat, fascia, and muscle remain unchanged. Over time, the added weight may exacerbate descent, blur contours, and distort facial proportions. The face may appear fuller, but not structurally younger.

The DeepFrame Facelift™ addresses this fundamental error by correcting the position of displaced tissues rather than masking their movement with volume. By restoring anatomy at its source, it resolves the apparent contradiction of simultaneous hollowing and heaviness that characterizes many aging faces.

One of the most significant advantages of structural repositioning lies in restoration of native contour. Youthful facial aesthetics are defined not by volume alone, but by the spatial arrangement of tissues relative to the skeleton. Smooth malar convexity, a short lid cheek junction, a defined jawline, and harmonious transitions between facial units all depend on proper positioning of existing tissues.

Fillers and fat grafts can soften hollows, but they cannot recreate the three dimensional curvature of the youthful face when underlying tissues have shifted. Added volume tends to expand outward from the point of injection, producing rounded or swollen contours that differ qualitatively from the smooth convexity created by properly positioned native tissue. This difference is subtle but perceptible, particularly in the midface and periorbital regions.

By repositioning existing fat compartments and soft tissue layers, the DeepFrame Facelift™ restores contour from within. The cheek regains projection by returning to its anatomical position rather than by being augmented. The lid cheek junction shortens as the cheek is elevated beneath the orbit rather than filled from below. Facial transitions become smooth because native tissues once again occupy their intended relationships. The result is fullness that appears inherent rather than added.

This distinction is critical for the preservation of facial identity. Augmentation tends to impose a generic fullness that can obscure individual skeletal characteristics. Structural repositioning reveals and restores those characteristics, allowing patients to look like themselves rather than like a volumized version of themselves.

Another important consideration is the cumulative effect of repeated volumetric treatments. Fillers and fat grafts are often promoted as temporary or reversible, yet in practice their effects can accumulate over time. Hyaluronic acid fillers may persist longer than expected, migrate from their original placement, or attract fluid through hydrophilic properties. Fat grafts introduce additional unpredictability related to survival, resorption, and potential hypertrophy.

As volumetric treatments are repeated to maintain effect or address new areas of concern, layers of material accumulate within tissue planes. This process can blur anatomical landmarks, distort natural contours, and create a heavy or amorphous appearance. In the periorbital region, even small amounts of excess volume can produce edema, irregularity, or impaired eyelid dynamics. In the lower face, fillers placed to camouflage jowls or pre jowl hollows may widen the jawline and undermine definition.

Cumulative distortion is not merely an aesthetic concern. It can complicate future surgical correction by obscuring tissue planes and altering anatomy. Dissection becomes more challenging, and outcomes become less predictable. Patients who have undergone extensive volumetric treatment often present with faces that are difficult to interpret anatomically, making structural correction more complex.

The DeepFrame Facelift™ avoids this cycle by addressing the cause of contour change rather than repeatedly compensating for its effects. Structural repositioning restores anatomy without introducing foreign material or additional mass. Tissue planes are preserved, and the face retains its natural architecture. When adjunctive volumization is indicated, it can be applied selectively within a corrected framework, minimizing the risk of cumulative distortion.

Longevity represents another area in which structural correction offers a clear advantage. Injectable fillers and fat grafts require repeated treatments to maintain effect. Their results are inherently temporary because they do not alter the structural forces driving aging. Each treatment addresses appearance at a single point in time without changing the trajectory of tissue descent. As gravity and mechanical load continue to act, hollows reappear, contours shift, and additional intervention becomes necessary.

In contrast, the DeepFrame Facelift™ produces a structural reset. By restoring deep support and repositioning tissues at their anatomical origin, it reduces the forces that cause visible aging. Midface elevation decreases inferior load on the lower face. Restoration of SMAS integrity stabilizes jawline contour. Reestablishment of platysmal continuity supports the neck. These changes alter the mechanical environment in which aging occurs.

Longevity is achieved not by resisting aging, but by restoring anatomy so that aging resumes from a corrected baseline. Changes occur more gradually and proportionately, and facial harmony is preserved over time. This distinction is essential for understanding why structural rejuvenation ages more gracefully than surface based or volumetric approaches.

Preservation of facial movement and expression further differentiates structural correction from volumetric augmentation. The face is a dynamic organ. Expression, speech, and emotional communication depend on coordinated movement of muscles within a balanced anatomical framework. Excessive volume in dynamic regions can interfere with this balance.

Overfilled faces often appear stiff, heavy, or emotionally blunted. This effect is particularly noticeable around the eyes and mouth, where subtle changes in contour or mobility have outsized impact on expression. Fillers placed beneath the lower eyelid may restrict movement or produce a puffy appearance that conveys fatigue rather than youth. Augmentation around the mouth can alter smile dynamics or create an unnatural fullness that draws attention to itself.

Because the DeepFrame Facelift™ relies on restoration rather than augmentation, it preserves normal muscle function and expressive nuance. Muscles operate within restored anatomical boundaries rather than against added mass. Skin redrapes over a supported framework rather than being stretched over injected volume. As a result, facial animation remains natural even as contour is improved.

Another advantage of structural correction is the reduction of long-term treatment burden. Patients who rely heavily on fillers or fat grafting often find themselves engaged in an ongoing cycle of maintenance. As aging progresses and results fade or distort, additional treatments are required. This cumulative burden can be costly, time-consuming, and emotionally taxing. Patients may feel trapped in a pattern of frequent interventions that produce diminishing returns.

Structural correction reduces dependence on repeated treatments by addressing the root cause of aging. While adjunctive procedures may still play a role, particularly for fine tuning or addressing true volume deficiency, they are used selectively rather than as primary corrective tools. This shift reduces overall intervention frequency and allows patients to enjoy longer periods of stability.

It is important to emphasize that the DeepFrame Facelift™ does not reject fillers or fat grafting outright. These modalities have a legitimate role when used judiciously and in appropriate contexts. True volume deficiency exists in some patients and in some regions. In such cases, volumetric augmentation can enhance results when applied within a structurally corrected framework.

The distinction lies in sequence and intent. Structural repositioning establishes the foundation. Volume is added only when necessary and only after anatomy has been restored. This approach avoids the pitfalls of compensatory volumization and allows fillers or fat grafts to function as refinements rather than crutches.

The contrast between volumetric camouflage and structural correction reflects a broader philosophical difference in facial rejuvenation. Superficial approaches focus on what appears deficient or irregular at the surface. Structural approaches ask why those appearances developed in the first place. By answering that question, the DeepFrame Facelift™ aligns intervention with anatomy rather than with visual symptom alone.

This alignment has important implications for long term tissue health. Injected materials alter tissue composition and may provoke inflammatory or fibrotic responses over time. While generally safe, their cumulative effects are not fully understood, particularly when used extensively or repeatedly over many years. Structural repositioning avoids introducing foreign substances or altering tissue composition, preserving the biological integrity of facial tissues.

From an aesthetic standpoint, the advantages of structural correction are cumulative and reinforcing. Restoration of midface position improves periorbital appearance. Stabilization of the lower face enhances neck contour. Each region benefits from the correction of adjacent regions, producing a cohesive result that cannot be replicated through isolated volumetric treatments.

In summary, fillers and fat grafting can provide meaningful improvement when used appropriately, but they are limited when applied as primary solutions for aging driven by structural displacement. By adding volume without restoring position, they risk cumulative distortion, interfere with natural movement, and require ongoing maintenance.

The DeepFrame Facelift™ offers a more durable and anatomically sound solution. By repositioning native tissues and restoring deep support, it recreates natural contour, preserves expression, and reduces long-term reliance on volumetric camouflage. This structural approach aligns rejuvenation with anatomy, providing a stable and harmonious foundation for facial aging to resume in a balanced and predictable manner.

CHAPTER 9

The Longevity of the DeepFrame Facelift™

Longevity is one of the most frequently discussed yet least clearly understood goals of facelift surgery. Patients often ask how long a facelift will last, but this question cannot be answered meaningfully without examining how aging occurs and how surgical correction interacts with that process. Longevity is not determined simply by the passage of time. It is determined by whether the intervention alters the mechanical environment that produces visible aging or merely compensates for its surface manifestations.[23,24]

Many facial rejuvenation procedures produce immediate visual improvement, yet their results deteriorate predictably. Skin loosens again, contours soften, and the appearance gradually returns toward its preoperative state. This pattern reflects the fact that surface-based corrections do not change the forces acting on facial tissues. When those forces remain unchanged, the outcome cannot be durable.

The DeepFrame Facelift™ is designed with longevity as a central objective. Its durability arises not from resisting aging, but from correcting the anatomical failures that allow aging to become visible. By restoring deep structural relationships and redistributing mechanical load, it alters the conditions under which aging proceeds. This distinction explains why structural rejuvenation produces results that persist and age gracefully rather than deteriorate abruptly.

To understand longevity in facelift surgery, it is necessary to view it as a biomechanical concept rather than a temporal one. Facial tissues exist within a dynamic mechanical system. They are subjected to gravity, muscular movement, and age related changes in skeletal and fascial support. When this system is disrupted, visible aging emerges. When it is restored, aging continues, but its visible effects are delayed and moderated.

Longevity in facial rejuvenation is therefore fundamentally biomechanical. Tissues that are required to bear sustained load will eventually stretch, deform, or fail. Skin and superficial fascia are particularly susceptible to this process. When correction relies on tightening these tissues, they must continuously oppose gravitational and muscular forces they are not designed to withstand. [23,24] Stretching, scar widening, and relapse are not complications in this context. They are predictable consequences of inappropriate load bearing.

Structural correction changes this equation. When tissues are repositioned to anatomically appropriate locations and supported by bone, deep fat, and robust fascial layers, the forces acting on them are reduced.[10,14,24] Load is redistributed to structures capable of maintaining it. Instead of resisting aging, the correction removes the conditions that accelerate visible aging. This shift in mechanics is the foundation of longevity.[23,24]

The DeepFrame Facelift™ applies this principle consistently across facial regions. Midface elevation restores support beneath the orbit and reduces inferior load. SMAS restoration stabilizes the lower face. Reestablishment of platysmal continuity supports the neck. Skin is allowed to redrape passively over this restored framework rather than serving as a primary support structure. [14,24] Each of these elements contributes to a more stable mechanical environment.

Many rejuvenation techniques provide temporary improvement without altering the underlying process of aging.[24,27] Fillers, skin tightening devices, and superficial lifts improve appearance at a single moment in time, but they do not change the direction or magnitude of tissue descent. They may mask aging, but they do not modify its cause.

The DeepFrame Facelift™ establishes what can be described as a structural reset. By restoring the position of the midface, reinforcing SMAS integrity, and reestablishing cervicofacial continuity, it creates a new anatomical baseline. From this baseline, aging resumes along a more favorable trajectory. The face does not remain frozen in a youthful state, but it ages from a position of restored balance rather than accumulated distortion.

This concept helps explain a phenomenon commonly observed after structural facelift surgery. Patients often report that they appear to age more slowly than before their procedure. In reality, aging continues at the same biological rate. What changes is the configuration from which aging proceeds. Because deep support has been restored, the visible effects of aging unfold more gradually and proportionately.

Vector alignment plays a critical role in this process. Aging occurs along predictable vectors determined by gravity, anatomy, and mechanical load. When corrective forces are applied along unnatural vectors, tissues are displaced in directions they are not designed to maintain. This mismatch places stress on fixation points and accelerates failure.

Corrections aligned with the original vectors of aging require less force to maintain position. They restore tissues along the same paths through which they descended, reversing displacement rather than redirecting it. This alignment reduces strain and enhances stability.

The DeepFrame Facelift™ restores tissues along vertical and oblique vectors that mirror the natural course of aging. Midface tissues are elevated vertically and anteriorly. Lower face tissues are repositioned along combined vertical and oblique vectors that restore jawline continuity. Cervical correction counters inferior and anterior descent without imposing excessive posterior tension. Because the direction of correction matches the direction of aging, the resulting anatomy is mechanically efficient and resistant to relapse.

Depth of correction is equally important. Superficial tissues stretch more readily and are more susceptible to age related degradation. Skin and superficial fascia are thin, elastic, and poorly suited for sustained load bearing. Deep tissues, particularly those anchored to bone or composed of dense fascia, provide far more durable support.

When correction is performed superficially, longevity is limited by the properties of the tissues being manipulated. When correction is performed deeply, longevity is governed by the stability of the anatomical framework.

The DeepFrame Facelift™ applies corrective forces at the depth appropriate to each anatomical problem. Sub-periosteal midface elevation restores malar support. SMAS manipulation stabilizes the lower face. Platysmal restoration reinforces the cervicofacial sling. Skin is redraped passively rather than tightened aggressively. This hierarchy of support ensures that load is borne by structures designed to maintain it.

Integration across facial regions further enhances longevity. Facial aging is a system-level process. Descent of the midface increases load on the lower face. Failure of lower face support accelerates cervical aging. Treating these regions independently creates competing forces that undermine durability.

Fragmented approaches may achieve localized improvement, but they often leave uncorrected forces that act against the repair. Over time, these forces erode results.

The DeepFrame Facelift™ integrates correction across the midface, lower face, and neck. By addressing inferior load at its source and coordinating vectors across regions, it distributes forces evenly throughout the cervicofacial complex. Each corrected region supports adjacent regions rather than opposing them. This integration is a critical contributor to long-term stability.

Longevity must also be understood in the context of what happens after structural correction. No surgical procedure halts aging. Skin continues to thin. Ligaments continue to attenuate. Skeletal remodeling progresses. These changes are unavoidable. What differs after structural rejuvenation is how these changes manifest.

When aging resumes from a corrected anatomical configuration, its visible effects are delayed and proportionate. Contours soften gradually rather than collapsing abruptly. Facial harmony is preserved even as subtle changes occur. Patients often describe looking consistently younger than their chronological age for many years, not because they appear unchanged, but because their faces remain balanced.

This distinction is essential. Longevity does not mean permanence. It means preservation of structure over time.

The role of surgical judgment in longevity cannot be overstated. Structural correction provides the framework for durable results, but it does not guarantee them automatically. Overcorrection can place undue stress on tissues and compromise longevity. Under correction leaves residual forces unaddressed. Misaligned vectors can create instability even when depth of correction is appropriate.

The DeepFrame Facelift™ requires careful anatomical assessment and individualized planning. The surgeon must determine which structures require correction, how aggressively to apply each maneuver, and how to balance competing forces across the face and neck. Longevity emerges from this synthesis rather than from adherence to a rigid protocol.

Patient-specific factors also influence durability. Tissue quality, skeletal anatomy, degree of aging, and lifestyle factors all play a role. Structural correction accommodates this variability better than superficial approaches because it adapts to anatomy rather than imposing a standardized solution.

It is also important to distinguish longevity from rigidity. A face that remains artificially tight for many years may appear durable in a narrow sense, but it does so at the cost of natural appearance. True longevity preserves natural movement and expression while maintaining structural coherence. The DeepFrame approach emphasizes this balance by restoring support without over-constraining dynamic tissues.

From a conceptual standpoint, longevity reflects alignment between surgical intervention and biological reality. Procedures that fight biology eventually lose. Procedures that restore anatomy work with biology rather than against it. The DeepFrame Facelift™ belongs to the latter category.

By reestablishing deep anatomical relationships, aligning corrective vectors with natural aging patterns, and integrating correction across facial regions, it alters the biomechanical environment in which aging occurs. Instead of accelerating visible aging through tension and distortion, it slows its appearance by restoring balance.

In summary, the longevity of the DeepFrame Facelift™ derives from its structural foundation. It does not rely on surface tension, volumetric camouflage, or isolated maneuvers. It restores the framework upon which youthful facial form depends. Aging continues, but it does so from a corrected baseline that preserves harmony, identity, and proportion.

This emphasis on biomechanical integrity distinguishes the DeepFrame approach from techniques that offer temporary improvement without lasting stability. It provides a meaningful and anatomically grounded answer to the question of longevity in facelift surgery and establishes structural restoration as the most reliable path to durable facial rejuvenation.

CHAPTER 10

The Advantages of the DeepFrame Facelift™ Over Other Facelift Techniques

Facelift surgery has evolved through multiple conceptual phases, each shaped by the prevailing understanding of facial aging at the time. Early techniques viewed aging primarily as a surface phenomenon, while later approaches progressively acknowledged the role of deeper structures such as fascia, muscle, and fat. More recent methods have attempted to mobilize composite tissue layers in pursuit of greater durability and more natural results. Despite this evolution, significant differences remain in how comprehensively various facelift techniques address aging as a structural and biomechanical process.

The DeepFrame Facelift™ distinguishes itself not as a variation on a single maneuver or plane of dissection, but as an integrated structural system. Its advantages over other facelift techniques arise from how it conceptualizes facial aging, how it distributes corrective forces, and how it integrates facial regions into a cohesive biomechanical framework. Rather than competing with existing techniques on the basis of access or branding, it represents a synthesis that resolves the limitations inherent in more narrowly defined approaches.

Understanding these advantages requires examining how other facelift techniques address aging and where their conceptual constraints limit outcomes.

Early facelift techniques focused almost exclusively on the skin. Aging was understood as laxity of the cutaneous envelope, and correction consisted of excision and redraping under tension. These approaches could produce immediate tightening and smoothing, but their shortcomings were predictable. Skin is not designed to bear sustained mechanical load.[3,5] When tension is placed on the skin as a primary support mechanism, it stretches over time. Scars widen, contours soften, and results deteriorate as underlying descent continues uncorrected.

Limited access techniques represent a modern extension of this surface-focused philosophy. By reducing incision length or dissection extent, they aim to minimize recovery while offering visible improvement. While appealing in concept, these approaches necessarily sacrifice depth of correction and vector accuracy. Improvements tend to be modest and short-lived, particularly in patients with significant midface descent, SMAS elongation, or cervical laxity. Because the underlying structural failures remain unaddressed, relapse is not a complication but an expected outcome.

The DeepFrame Facelift™ avoids these limitations by relocating corrective forces away from the skin and into deep tissues capable of maintaining support. Skin redraping is treated as a secondary step that reflects restored structure rather than as a primary means of correction. This shift fundamentally alters both the appearance and durability of results.

Recognition of the limitations of skin-based techniques led to the development of SMAS plication and imbrication procedures. These methods represented an important conceptual advance by acknowledging the role of the superficial musculoaponeurotic system in facial aging. By tightening or folding this fascial layer, surgeons were able to improve support relative to skin only approaches and reduce reliance on cutaneous tension.

However, older SMAS plication techniques often treat the SMAS as a uniform structure and rely heavily on lateral vectors of correction. This assumption overlooks regional variability in SMAS thickness, strength, and contribution to aging. In many patients, SMAS elongation is not uniform, and displacement of deep tissues cannot be corrected adequately through plication alone.

More importantly, oblique SMAS plication does not address aging at the level of skeletal attachment.[4,5] Midface descent, infraorbital retrusion, and maxillary remodeling remain largely uncorrected. While jawline contour may improve initially, unaddressed midface descent continues to transmit load into the lower face and neck.[2,4,6] Over time, this undermines durability and limits the global rejuvenation effect.

The DeepFrame Facelift™ incorporates SMAS elevation where appropriate and SMAS plication in other patients who benefit from this maneuver. However, it does so as one component of a broader structural system, and in either case utilizes vectors more appropriately than older procedures. SMAS reinforcement or mobilization is applied selectively based on regional anatomy and degree of failure. It is integrated with subperiosteal midface elevation and coordinated cervical support, ensuring that correction occurs at the depth where aging originates rather than being confined to a single fascial layer.

Traditional deep plane facelifts represent a further evolution toward deeper correction. By elevating the skin and SMAS as a composite flap, these techniques reduce skin tension. Longevity is generally improved, and the risk of a pulled appearance can be reduced.

Despite these strengths, many deep plane techniques remain limited by their reliance on relatively uniform vectors and a single plane of dissection. While composite elevation can indirectly influence the midface, it often does not achieve true repositioning at the level of skeletal attachment.[3,7] Composite lifts suffer from single vector mobility of both the skin and the SMAS, though the aging process of these layers differs dramatically. Midface elevation may be incomplete or dependent on lateral traction rather than vertical restoration.

Additionally, deep plane dissection alone does not address skeletal remodeling or allow fine control of region-specific vectors. Aging does not occur at a uniform depth across the face, and a single plane approach risks overcorrecting some regions while undercorrecting others. The result may be improvement without optimal balance or durability.

The DeepFrame Facelift™ builds upon the conceptual strengths of deep plane surgery while extending them into a more anatomically complete system. It employs multiple planes of correction tailored to regional anatomy and aging patterns. Subperiosteal elevation restores midface support at the skeletal interface. SMAS manipulation stabilizes the lower face. Platysmal continuity is restored to support the neck. Each maneuver is selected based on the specific structural failure being addressed rather than adherence to a single access strategy.

Isolated subperiosteal midface lifts illustrate the importance of integration in facial rejuvenation. When performed alone, subperiosteal elevation can effectively restore cheek position and periorbital support. However, if lower face and neck correction are not coordinated, imbalance may result. The midface may appear elevated above a descended jawline or unsupported neck, creating discordance rather than harmony.

The DeepFrame Facelift™ integrates subperiosteal midface elevation into a comprehensive cervicofacial strategy. By addressing the midface, lower face, and neck as interdependent regions, it prevents competing forces and ensures that improvements in one area reinforce, rather than undermine, results elsewhere. This integration enhances both aesthetic coherence and longevity.

One of the most significant advantages of the DeepFrame Facelift™ over other techniques is its emphasis on vector integration. Facial aging occurs along predictable vectors determined by gravity, ligamentous attenuation, and mechanical load. Techniques that rely on uniform lateral traction or excessive tightening often apply forces that do not align with these natural patterns.

Misaligned vectors place stress on fixation points and tissues, accelerating relapse and contributing to distortion. They may also alter facial proportions by widening the face or flattening natural curvature.

The DeepFrame approach restores tissues along region-specific vectors that mirror their original descent. Vertical and superolateral vectors restore midface position. Composite vertical and oblique vectors correct the lower face. Superolateral and vertical support stabilize the neck. This alignment reduces mechanical stress, improves stability, and preserves natural facial proportions.

Adaptability to individual anatomy represents another important advantage. Many facelift techniques are defined by standardized maneuvers that are applied similarly across patients. While this consistency may simplify teaching or marketing, it limits adaptability. Facial skeletons vary widely. Soft tissue thickness, ligamentous integrity, and aging patterns differ from patient to patient.

The DeepFrame Facelift™ functions as a framework rather than a formula. It provides principles for decision-making rather than a rigid sequence of steps. Surgeons assess which anatomical layers require correction, which planes offer the most effective access, and which vectors best restore balance. This adaptability allows the procedure to be tailored to diverse anatomies while maintaining a coherent structural philosophy.

Preservation of facial identity and expression is a critical consideration in evaluating facelift techniques. Approaches that rely heavily on tension, uniform vectors, or volumetric augmentation risk imposing an external aesthetic template on the patient. While such results may appear technically successful, they can subtly alter facial character and expression.

The DeepFrame Facelift™ prioritizes restoration rather than reshaping. By returning tissues toward their pre-aging anatomical positions, it preserves the patient's inherent skeletal structure, soft tissue distribution, and expressive patterns. Muscles operate within restored anatomical boundaries rather than against imposed constraints. The face remains recognizable, and expression remains dynamic.

Durability further distinguishes structural approaches from technique-driven ones. Facelift longevity is not simply a function of surgical access or extent of dissection. It reflects how effectively the procedure redistributes mechanical load and restores support at appropriate depths. Techniques that rely on superficial correction inevitably deteriorate as tissues stretch and forces persist.

By restoring deep anatomical relationships and integrating correction across facial regions, the DeepFrame Facelift™ alters the biomechanical environment in which aging occurs. Load is reduced rather than resisted. Tension is distributed to structures capable of maintaining it. As a result, outcomes age more gracefully and predictably.

It is also important to recognize that the DeepFrame approach does not reject other techniques outright. Many elements of existing facelifts contribute meaningfully to its framework. Skin redraping, SMAS manipulation, deep plane mobilization, and subperiosteal elevation each have a role. The distinction lies in how these elements are integrated and applied.

Rather than offering a competing technique, the DeepFrame Facelift™ represents an evolution toward anatomically complete facial rejuvenation. It resolves the limitations of earlier methods by addressing aging as a multi-layer, multi-vector, and system-level process.

In summary, the advantages of the DeepFrame Facelift™ over other facelift techniques derive from its structural philosophy. By addressing aging at multiple anatomical levels, aligning corrective vectors with true aging patterns, and integrating correction across the cervicofacial complex, it achieves natural appearance, mechanical stability, and long-term durability.

Rather than focusing on access, or isolated maneuvers, the DeepFrame approach provides a comprehensive framework for understanding and correcting facial aging. It reflects a maturation of facelift surgery from technique-driven intervention toward anatomically grounded structural restoration and offers a durable, adaptable, and identity-preserving path to facial rejuvenation.

CHAPTER 11

Surgical Planning, Customization, and Intraoperative Decision Making

Structural facial rejuvenation cannot be reduced to a fixed sequence of operative steps because faces do not age according to a uniform biological script. Although many facelift techniques are described as reproducible formulas, aging itself is neither standardized nor predictable in its expression. The magnitude, direction, and depth of tissue change vary between individuals and even between regions of the same face. For this reason, any approach that relies on a rigid protocol risks either undercorrecting the true source of aging or introducing distortion by applying correction where it is not anatomically indicated. The DeepFrame Facelift™ was conceived specifically to address this variability. It functions not as a predefined operation but as a structural system that guides planning, execution, and intraoperative decision making according to anatomy and biomechanics rather than predetermined steps.

At the core of the DeepFrame philosophy is the understanding that surgical planning is inseparable from diagnosis. Planning does not begin with deciding which incisions to make or which plane to enter, but with identifying the anatomical failures that have produced the patient's current appearance. Surface findings such as folds, laxity, or asymmetry are considered consequences rather than causes. Effective planning therefore requires a comprehensive assessment of skeletal support, deep fat compartment position, ligamentous integrity, fascial behavior, muscular dynamics, and the way in which load is transmitted across the face and neck. This assessment establishes the framework within which surgical decisions are made.

Preoperative evaluation in the DeepFrame approach extends beyond static visual inspection. Dynamic observation during facial expression reveals how muscles interact with overlying soft tissues and whether motion is constrained or exaggerated by underlying laxity. Skeletal landmarks are assessed not as targets for alteration, but as reference points that define the original architecture of the face. The surgeon must determine how far tissues have migrated from these reference points and which layers have failed to maintain their supportive role.

Midface position is a central focus of this analysis because it influences nearly every other region of the face. The relationship between the cheek and the orbit affects lower eyelid contour and lid cheek junction length. Inferior displacement of the midface increases load on the lower face and accelerates jowl formation. Uncorrected midface descent compromises the durability of lower face and neck correction regardless of how aggressively those regions are treated. Surgical planning therefore begins with understanding whether midface displacement is present, how severe it is, and whether it must be addressed at the level of skeletal attachment to achieve meaningful correction.

The lower face is evaluated in the context of SMAS behavior rather than skin laxity.[5,9,14] Jowls are interpreted as evidence of SMAS elongation and medial migration of soft tissues rather than as redundant skin.[5,9,22] The mandibular border is assessed as a structural boundary whose clarity or definition depends on deep support rather than superficial tightening. [21,22] Similarly, the neck is examined as the inferior extension of the cervicofacial support system. Platysmal behavior, cervical contour, and cervicomental angle are evaluated in relation to lower face and midface position rather than as isolated aesthetic concerns.

Asymmetries are interpreted carefully, with the understanding that some asymmetry is congenital and normal, while other facial asymmetry reflects differential descent. One side of the face often demonstrates greater ligamentous attenuation or skeletal retrusion, leading to uneven aging. Recognizing this distinction is essential for planning asymmetric correction that restores balance without forcing symmetry.

Vector planning represents an area in which preoperative analysis and intraoperative judgment converge. Aging follows predictable directional patterns dictated by gravity, anatomy, and biomechanical load. However, the degree to which tissues respond to correction varies based on tissue quality, elasticity, and prior intervention. Preoperative planning establishes an initial vector strategy based on anatomical analysis, but true refinement occurs intraoperatively as tissues are mobilized and observed.

Intraoperative assessment allows the surgeon to evaluate how tissues move when released, how much force is required to reposition them, and where that force is best supported. Vectors are adjusted to ensure that elevation follows anatomically appropriate paths and that load is transferred to deep, durable structures rather than superficial tissues. The objective is biomechanical efficiency rather than maximal elevation. Correction that requires excessive force is inherently unstable. Correction that aligns with natural vectors of aging requires less force and maintains its position more reliably.

The integration of vectors across regions is central to the DeepFrame approach. Elevation of the midface reduces inferior forces acting on the lower face. Restoration of SMAS support decreases strain transmitted to the platysma. When vectors are coordinated, corrective forces reinforce one another and create a balanced structural system. When vectors compete, stress accumulates at fixation points and relapse becomes more likely. Surgical planning therefore considers the face as a unified biomechanical entity rather than a collection of independent aesthetic units.

Attention to neurovascular anatomy is fundamental throughout the procedure. Structural facelift surgery requires precise dissection within defined anatomical planes to preserve facial nerve branches and maintain adequate vascular supply. The DeepFrame approach emphasizes respect for these structures over aggressive correction. Dissection depth and extent are adjusted based on individual anatomical variation, prior surgical history, and tissue quality. Preservation of perfusion and nerve integrity is not merely a safety consideration, but a determinant of aesthetic quality and longevity. Compromised vascularity impairs healing and scar quality. Nerve injury alters expression and undermines the very identity the procedure seeks to preserve.

Skin management in the DeepFrame Facelift™ reflects the principle that skin is a covering rather than a support structure. Skin is addressed only after deep plane correction has been completed. Once underlying tissues have been repositioned and supported, the skin is allowed to redrape naturally over the restored framework. Excess skin is excised conservatively, guided by natural drape rather than tension. This sequence ensures that the skin reflects underlying anatomy rather than compensates for its absence. Low tension closure improves scar quality, preserves vascularity, and reduces the risk of distortion or pulled appearance.

Intraoperative restraint is a defining characteristic of the DeepFrame philosophy. Structural correction does not require maximal tightening, exaggerated elevation, or uniform correction across all regions. Overcorrection can be as detrimental as undercorrection. Excessive elevation distorts proportions and compromises function. Excessive tightening places load on tissues not designed to bear it. The surgeon's task is to recognize when anatomical relationships have been adequately restored and to resist the impulse to pursue additional change simply because it is technically possible.

Balance and harmony guide intraoperative decision making. Symmetry is evaluated dynamically rather than statically, with the understanding that perfect symmetry is neither achievable nor desirable. The relationship between regions is continually reassessed to confirm that correction in one area supports rather than destabilizes adjacent areas. The endpoint of the procedure is reached when the face appears structurally coherent and when tension has been transferred to deep, durable tissues capable of maintaining support over time.

The flexibility inherent in the DeepFrame Facelift™ resists commoditization. Because the procedure is not defined by a rigid protocol, its success depends on anatomical knowledge, judgment, and experience. This reliance on surgical reasoning is not a limitation, but a strength. It allows the procedure to accommodate the wide variability of human facial anatomy and aging patterns while maintaining a consistent structural philosophy. The DeepFrame approach cannot be reduced to a checklist or taught as a single maneuver. It must be understood as a system of decisions guided by anatomy and biomechanics.

In this way, surgical planning and intraoperative decision making are not ancillary considerations, but central components of the DeepFrame Facelift™. The procedure achieves its results not through standardized execution, but through thoughtful customization that restores deep support while preserving safety, function, and identity. By tailoring planes of correction, vectors, and extent of intervention to the individual patient, the DeepFrame approach produces rejuvenation that is anatomically coherent, mechanically stable, and durable over time.

CHAPTER 12

Recovery, Healing, and the Evolution of Results Over Time

Understanding recovery is inseparable from understanding outcome in structural facial rejuvenation. Unlike superficial aesthetic interventions that aim to produce an immediate visual change, a structurally based facelift initiates a sequence of anatomical, biomechanical, and biological events that unfold gradually over time. The DeepFrame Facelift™ does not produce a single static result that appears fully formed in the early postoperative period. Instead, it establishes a corrected anatomical framework within which healing, adaptation, and long term refinement occur. The final aesthetic outcome is therefore not a moment, but a process.

This distinction is fundamental. Many misconceptions about facelift recovery arise from the assumption that surgical rejuvenation should be judged in the early weeks after surgery. In reality, early postoperative appearance reflects swelling, tissue response, and temporary changes in neuromuscular behavior rather than the true result of structural correction. The DeepFrame Facelift™

is intentionally designed to support predictable healing and progressive refinement by placing correction in deep, stable tissues and minimizing reliance on skin tension or superficial fixation. As a result, recovery follows a biologically coherent trajectory that mirrors the restoration of anatomy rather than the forced manipulation of appearance.

In the immediate postoperative period, the most prominent features are swelling, bruising, and a sense of tightness or stiffness. These findings are expected and reflect normal inflammatory response to surgical intervention. Because the DeepFrame approach involves mobilization and repositioning of deep plane tissues, early edema may appear more diffuse than after procedures that focus primarily on the skin. This swelling does not indicate excessive trauma. Rather, it reflects the physiological response of deeper tissue planes as they adapt to restored position and altered load distribution.

A critical difference between structural and superficial techniques becomes apparent even at this early stage. Because the DeepFrame Facelift™ does not rely on skin tension to maintain correction, the early postoperative face rarely appears pulled, distorted, or over tightened. Facial proportions remain recognizable, and the relationship between facial regions is preserved despite swelling. The patient's identity is maintained, even before refinement has occurred. This preservation of proportion and identity is not incidental. It reflects the fact that correction has been achieved by restoring support rather than by imposing tension.

Neurological function during the early postoperative period is typically preserved. Temporary changes in sensation or movement may occur due to swelling, but these resolve progressively as inflammation subsides. Because facial nerve branches are respected and dissection is performed within defined anatomical planes, functional recovery follows a predictable course. Facial expression gradually returns as swelling diminishes, and dynamic movement is not constrained by excessive skin tightening or superficial fixation.

As the early inflammatory phase resolves over the first several weeks, the recovery process enters a period of transition. Edema decreases, bruising fades, and tissues begin to settle into their restored positions. During this phase, the benefits of structural correction become increasingly apparent. The jawline sharpens as jowl tissue remains elevated within the cheek rather than migrating inferiorly. Cervical definition improves as platysmal support stabilizes and inferior load from the face has been reduced. Midface projection becomes more consistent as repositioned tissues adapt to their skeletal foundation.

Importantly, changes observed during this intermediate phase reflect refinement rather than relapse. Because correction has been anchored in deep planes, tissues are not dependent on skin tension to maintain position. As swelling resolves, the face does not collapse or descend. Instead, contours become clearer and transitions between facial units soften naturally. The appearance becomes progressively more natural rather than more artificial with time.

Scar maturation also begins during this period. Low tension closure and respect for vascularity promote favorable scar quality. Incisions soften and blend into surrounding tissue as collagen remodeling occurs. Because skin has not been used as a load bearing structure, scar widening and distortion are minimized. This contributes not only to aesthetic outcome, but also to patient comfort and confidence during recovery.

Between approximately three and six months after surgery, healing enters a phase of structural integration. This phase is critical to the long term success of the DeepFrame Facelift™ and represents the point at which the procedure's structural philosophy is fully realized. Fascial layers remodel in their new positions. Fixation points strengthen as biological healing reinforces surgical correction. Soft tissues adapt to restored anatomical relationships and establish new patterns of load transmission.

During this phase, the face increasingly appears not surgically altered, but structurally restored. Facial harmony improves as transitions between aesthetic units become smooth and proportional. The lid cheek junction appears shorter and more youthful because midface position has been restored rather than filled.[2,4] The mandibular border appears clean and continuous because deep support has been reestablished. Cervical contour appears natural and integrated with the lower face rather than sharply separated or artificially tightened.

Expression during this period remains dynamic and unforced. Because muscles and skin are not constrained by excessive tension, facial animation occurs within restored anatomical boundaries. The patient looks like themselves, but refreshed. This quality is often described by patients as appearing rested or healthier rather than altered. From a structural perspective, this reflects the fact that the face is functioning within a corrected biomechanical environment rather than compensating for ongoing structural failure.

The concept of a corrected baseline is central to understanding long term outcome. No surgical procedure halts the biological processes of aging. Skin continues to thin. Ligaments continue to attenuate. Skeletal remodeling progresses gradually over time. However, when aging resumes from a corrected anatomical configuration, its visible effects are delayed and distributed more evenly. The face ages from a position of restored balance rather than from a state of advanced displacement.

Over the long term, patients who undergo the DeepFrame Facelift™ typically experience slower recurrence of jowling, better preservation of cervical definition, and sustained improvement in periorbital support. These observations are not the result of resisting aging, but of having reduced the mechanical forces that accelerate visible aging. By restoring midface position, inferior load on the lower face and neck is reduced. By reinforcing SMAS support, strain on superficial tissues is minimized. By maintaining cervicofacial continuity, the neck ages in concert with the face rather than as an isolated region.

Patients often report that they continue to look younger than their peers for many years following surgery, even as they continue to age. This perception reflects preservation of facial harmony rather than static appearance. The face continues to change, but it does so in a manner that remains proportionate and coherent. This distinction is central to the concept of longevity discussed in earlier chapters and is reinforced by the recovery trajectory itself.

Adjunctive treatments may still play a role after structural correction, but their function is fundamentally altered. Skin quality continues to evolve with age, sun exposure, and environmental factors. Selective use of resurfacing, neuromodulators, or limited volumization may enhance surface appearance or address isolated concerns. However, these treatments function as refinements rather than primary corrective tools. The structural foundation established by the DeepFrame Facelift™ reduces dependence on repeated volumetric camouflage or aggressive skin tightening.

This shift has practical implications for patients. The cumulative treatment burden is reduced. Interventions become more targeted and less frequent. The risk of cumulative distortion from repeated filler or fat grafting is minimized. Future treatments, if desired, are performed on tissues that retain their anatomical clarity rather than being obscured by prior volumization.

Recovery also encompasses psychological adaptation. As swelling resolves and results stabilize, patients often experience a renewed alignment between how they feel internally and how they appear externally. This alignment is an important but often overlooked aspect of outcome. When facial rejuvenation preserves identity and expression, psychological adaptation tends to be positive and affirming. Patients recognize themselves in the mirror, but perceive a version that reflects vitality rather than fatigue or decline.

Because the DeepFrame approach avoids exaggeration and distortion, this adaptation is rarely disorienting. Patients do not feel that their appearance has been imposed upon them. Instead, they experience restoration of features they associate with their own facial identity. This contributes to long term satisfaction and confidence, and reinforces the importance of structural rather than superficial correction.

In contrast, procedures that rely heavily on surface tension or volumetric camouflage often produce early visual change that deteriorates over time. Initial tightness following other procedures can give way to stretching. Inappropriately added volume migrates or accumulates. Distortion becomes more apparent if unsupported tissues continue to age beneath uncorrected structural failure. Recovery in these cases may appear rapid, but long term evolution is often disappointing.

The DeepFrame Facelift™ reverses this pattern. Early recovery emphasizes healing rather than display. Intermediate recovery emphasizes refinement rather than correction. Long term evolution emphasizes stability rather than maintenance. Each phase reinforces the structural logic of the procedure and validates its underlying philosophy.

Ultimately, recovery after the DeepFrame Facelift™ is not simply the resolution of surgical effects, but the gradual realization of anatomical restoration. The procedure initiates a process in which tissues heal, integrate, and adapt to a corrected framework. The result is not frozen youth, but durable rejuvenation that ages gracefully over time.

This evolution of results underscores the central principle of the DeepFrame approach. Lasting facial rejuvenation does not arise from forcing appearance or resisting biology. It arises from restoring anatomy in a way that allows biology to proceed from a healthier, more balanced starting point.

CHAPTER 13

Safety, Risk Management, and Complication Avoidance in Structural Facelift Surgery

Any comprehensive discussion of facial rejuvenation must address safety with the same depth, rigor, and intellectual honesty applied to aesthetics and longevity. In facelift surgery, safety is often framed narrowly as the avoidance of specific complications, yet this perspective is incomplete. True surgical safety is not merely the absence of adverse events, but the predictable preservation of function, vascularity, identity, and long term tissue health. In structural facelift surgery, safety is inseparable from anatomy, biomechanics, and judgment.

The DeepFrame Facelift™ operates within this broader definition of safety. Although it involves deeper anatomical planes than superficial techniques, it does not increase risk when performed within a disciplined anatomical framework. In many respects, it reduces risk by minimizing skin tension, preserving vascular integrity, redistributing mechanical load to appropriate structures, and avoiding the compensatory maneuvers that often generate complications in surface based approaches. Structural correction, when guided by anatomical precision and restraint, is not inherently more dangerous than superficial correction. It is frequently safer.

Understanding why this is true requires reframing safety as an anatomical and biomechanical concept rather than a procedural one. Complications in facelift surgery most often arise when anatomy is violated, when tissues are placed under forces they are not designed to bear, or when correction is applied indiscriminately rather than selectively. Each of these failure modes is directly addressed by the structural philosophy of the DeepFrame Facelift™.

Facial anatomy is organized into predictable layers, each with distinct mechanical properties, vascular supply, and functional roles. Safety depends on respecting these layers and working within established planes rather than against them. When dissection strays from known anatomical boundaries, the risk of nerve injury, vascular compromise, and tissue ischemia increases. When correction relies on surface tension rather than deep support, the risk of skin necrosis, scarring, distortion, and relapse rises. When maneuvers are standardized rather than tailored, the likelihood of overcorrection or functional impairment grows.

The DeepFrame Facelift™ is intentionally designed to mitigate these risks by restoring anatomy rather than forcing appearance. Its safety profile emerges not from avoidance of depth, but from disciplined engagement with it.

Facial nerve preservation is a central concern in any facelift procedure and assumes heightened importance in structural approaches that engage deeper planes. The facial nerve and its branches follow consistent anatomical courses, but their depth and relationship to surrounding structures vary by region. Injury risk increases when dissection is blind, when traction is excessive, or when tissue resistance is overcome by force rather than release.

The DeepFrame approach emphasizes controlled dissection within defined planes and minimizes blind traction. Tissues are mobilized through anatomical release rather than aggressive pulling. This distinction is critical. When tissues are released at their points of fixation, they can be repositioned with minimal force. When release is inadequate and elevation is attempted through traction, force is transmitted to structures that should not bear it, including nerve branches.

By restoring mobility at the level of pathology, the DeepFrame Facelift™ reduces the need for forceful manipulation. This reduces strain on nerve branches and lowers the likelihood of neuropraxia. Preservation of facial nerve function is therefore not achieved by avoiding depth, but by avoiding tension and respecting anatomy. When correction is accomplished through release and repositioning rather than traction, nerve safety is enhanced rather than compromised.

Equally important is preservation of vascular supply. Skin flap viability depends on maintenance of the subdermal plexus and avoidance of excessive tension that can compromise perfusion. Historically, skin necrosis has been associated with aggressive skin undermining combined with high tension redraping, particularly in smokers or patients with compromised vascularity.[5] These risks are exacerbated when skin is asked to serve as a structural support rather than a covering layer.

In the DeepFrame Facelift™, skin is deliberately removed from the role of load bearing structure. Deep tissues carry the mechanical correction, and skin is redraped passively over restored anatomy. Because tension is minimal, perfusion is preserved. This approach promotes reliable healing even in patients with thinner skin, prior surgical scars, or borderline vascular risk factors. Rather than relying on robust skin to tolerate tension, the procedure minimizes the need for skin to tolerate stress at all.

This principle has downstream effects on multiple safety domains. Reduced skin tension improves scar quality and lowers the risk of wound healing complications. Incisions are closed under low strain, which supports favorable collagen remodeling and reduces the likelihood of widening, distortion, or hypertrophy. Scar placement can be optimized for concealment rather than mechanical necessity. Over time, scars soften and integrate more naturally into surrounding tissue.

Hematoma remains one of the most common early complications of facelift surgery and is influenced by multiple factors including blood pressure control, meticulous hemostasis, and postoperative management. Structural correction does not inherently increase hematoma risk. In fact, by avoiding excessive skin undermining and reducing tension on vascular structures, the DeepFrame approach may reduce mechanical stress on small vessels that contribute to postoperative bleeding.

Dead space management is also influenced by structural philosophy. When tissues are repositioned and supported in deep planes, potential spaces are reduced and tissue apposition is improved. This can decrease the likelihood of fluid accumulation and seroma formation. As with any surgical procedure, careful intraoperative hemostasis and vigilant postoperative monitoring remain essential, but structural correction does not introduce unique hematoma risks when executed properly.

Another important aspect of safety is avoidance of overcorrection. Overcorrection is not a benign aesthetic error. It can lead to functional impairment, distortion of facial expression, and increased complication risk. Excessive tightening can impair eyelid closure, alter oral commissure position, restrict cervical movement, and create unnatural facial proportions. These outcomes are often the result of equating surgical success with maximal visible change rather than anatomical normalization.

The DeepFrame philosophy explicitly rejects this approach. Correction is considered complete when anatomical relationships are restored, not when maximal elevation has been achieved. This restraint is not conservative in the sense of doing less, but disciplined in the sense of doing what is necessary and no more. By restoring structure rather than exaggerating form, the procedure protects both appearance and function.

This emphasis on restraint also enhances safety in dynamic regions such as the lower face and neck, where excessive tightening can interfere with speech, mastication, swallowing, or head movement. By placing corrective forces in deep, stable tissues and allowing superficial layers to move freely, the DeepFrame approach preserves functional range of motion while restoring contour.

Patient specific factors play a critical role in risk management and must be incorporated into surgical planning. Smoking status, vascular disease, connective tissue quality, prior surgery, and systemic health conditions all influence healing capacity and complication risk. Structural principles do not mandate aggressive intervention. They provide a framework within which intervention can be scaled appropriately.

The DeepFrame Facelift™ is inherently adaptable. The extent and depth of correction can be modified to balance benefit and risk in each individual patient. In some cases, limited deep correction may be combined with conservative surface refinement. In others, comprehensive structural restoration may be appropriate. Safety is enhanced when the procedure is tailored rather than standardized.

Revision facelift surgery presents unique safety challenges due to altered anatomy, scar tissue, and compromised vascularity. In these cases, structural understanding becomes even more important. Superficial revision techniques may temporarily improve appearance but often perpetuate the underlying structural deficiencies that led to relapse. Carefully planned structural correction can restore deep support and improve durability, but must be executed with heightened caution.

In revision settings, the DeepFrame approach emphasizes conservative dissection, preservation of remaining vascular supply, and avoidance of excessive correction. Anatomical landmarks may be distorted, and nerve branches may be more vulnerable. Surgical judgment and experience are paramount. When approached thoughtfully, structural correction can be performed safely and effectively even in complex revision cases.

It is important to recognize that safety is not achieved through avoidance of complexity, but through mastery of it. Structural facelift surgery requires deeper anatomical knowledge and greater technical precision than superficial techniques. However, this complexity serves a purpose. By addressing aging at its source and restoring normal biomechanics, the procedure reduces the need for compensatory maneuvers that generate risk.

In this sense, the DeepFrame Facelift™ represents a convergence of innovation and conservatism. It is innovative in its integration of multiple planes, vector coordination, and biomechanical reasoning. It is conservative in its respect for anatomy, its avoidance of unnecessary tension, and its emphasis on restoration rather than exaggeration.

When viewed through this lens, safety is not an adjunct consideration, but a direct outcome of structural philosophy. By working within anatomical planes, preserving neurovascular integrity, minimizing skin tension, and exercising restraint, the DeepFrame approach achieves a high margin of safety alongside its aesthetic and longevity advantages.

Ultimately, complication avoidance in facelift surgery is not about eliminating risk entirely, which is neither realistic nor honest. It is about understanding where risk arises and designing surgical strategy to minimize it without compromising outcome. The DeepFrame Facelift™ accomplishes this by aligning surgical correction with anatomy and biomechanics rather than forcing tissues to conform to surface ideals.

When performed within its anatomical framework by an experienced surgeon, the DeepFrame Facelift™ offers not only durable and natural rejuvenation, but also a robust safety profile. Structural restoration, guided by judgment and restraint, is not more dangerous than superficial correction. In many cases, it is safer.

CHAPTER 14

Outcomes, Satisfaction, and the Long Term Patient Experience

The success of facial rejuvenation cannot be meaningfully judged by early postoperative photographs or by isolated aesthetic changes observed in the weeks following surgery. While initial appearance matters, it represents only a small fraction of what patients ultimately experience. True success in facelift surgery is defined by durability, preservation of identity, functional integrity, and the way the result integrates into the patient's life over time. Structural approaches such as the DeepFrame Facelift™ are specifically designed to optimize these broader and more consequential measures of outcome by restoring anatomy rather than imposing surface change.

Patients do not live in static images. They live in motion, expression, social interaction, and gradual aging. Outcomes must therefore be evaluated in dynamic, longitudinal terms. The DeepFrame Facelift™ was developed with this perspective in mind. Its goal is not to produce a dramatic moment, but to establish a stable anatomical foundation that supports natural appearance, confidence, and satisfaction for years after surgery.

Aesthetic outcomes following the DeepFrame Facelift™ are characterized by global facial harmony rather than isolated improvement in a single region. Because correction is applied at the structural level and coordinated across the midface, lower face, and neck, changes occur in concert. Elevation of the midface restores periorbital support and cheek contour. Reinforcement of the SMAS redefines the jawline. Cervical correction refines the neck and cervicomental angle. Each improvement reinforces the others, producing a cohesive result that appears anatomically coherent rather than surgically constructed.

This integration is critical. Many facelift techniques produce localized improvement that draws attention to what has changed. A sharpened jawline paired with persistent midface descent or a smooth neck beneath an untreated lower face can create visual discordance. In contrast, structural rejuvenation produces proportional change. Transitions between aesthetic units remain smooth. Facial curvature is restored rather than exaggerated. The face appears balanced, rested, and internally consistent.

Patients frequently describe the outcome not in technical terms, but experiential ones. They report looking healthier, more energetic, or more like themselves at an earlier stage of life. Importantly, they rarely describe looking different. This distinction is central to satisfaction and reflects one of the most defining strengths of the DeepFrame approach.

Preservation of facial identity emerges consistently as one of the most valued outcomes. Identity in facial surgery is not an abstract concept. It is expressed through proportions, habitual expressions, and subtle asymmetries that make a face recognizable. Techniques that rely on uniform vectors, excessive tightening, or volumetric exaggeration risk overriding these features and replacing them with a generic aesthetic.

The DeepFrame Facelift™ avoids this outcome by restoring tissues toward their original anatomical positions rather than reshaping them according to an external ideal. Skeletal structure is respected. Native soft tissue distribution is preserved. Muscles operate within restored anatomical boundaries rather than against imposed tension. As a result, patients recognize themselves in the mirror. Friends and family often notice improvement without being able to identify a specific intervention.

This preservation of identity has significant psychological implications. When patients feel recognizable, the adjustment to their postoperative appearance is affirming rather than disorienting. They do not feel the need to explain or justify their appearance. Social interactions resume naturally, without anxiety about looking altered or artificial.

Functional outcomes are equally important and closely linked to patient satisfaction. The face is a dynamic structure involved in communication, nutrition, and emotional expression. Functional compromise, even when subtle, can undermine an otherwise successful aesthetic result.

Structural correction prioritizes function by placing corrective forces in deep, stable tissues rather than in skin or superficial fascia. Facial nerve integrity is preserved. Eyelid competence is maintained. Oral mobility remains unrestricted. Cervical movement is not constrained by excessive tension. Patients typically regain normal facial movement early in the recovery process, and expression remains fluid and authentic.

These functional outcomes contribute to a sense of ease in daily life. Patients do not feel stiff or constrained. Speech, mastication, and swallowing are unaffected. The face feels natural to inhabit, which reinforces long term satisfaction.

Durability is another critical dimension of outcome that is best assessed over time rather than in the early postoperative period. Patients who undergo the DeepFrame Facelift™ often report that their appearance remains stable for many years, with changes occurring gradually rather than abruptly. The face continues to age, but it does so from a corrected anatomical baseline.

This pattern is particularly evident in regions that are prone to early relapse after superficial procedures. Jowls recur more slowly because SMAS support has been restored and inferior load from the midface has been reduced.[5,6] Neck definition persists longer because cervicofacial continuity has been reestablished rather than masked. Periorbital support remains improved because the cheek has been repositioned beneath the eyelid.

Patients often describe a sustained sense of looking younger than their chronological age rather than a fleeting postoperative improvement. This perception reflects preservation of facial harmony rather than maintenance of a fixed appearance. Aging continues, but its visible effects are delayed and proportionate.

The reduced need for ongoing maintenance procedures is a meaningful contributor to long term satisfaction. Patients who have relied heavily on fillers, skin tightening, or other non structural interventions often describe a cycle of repeated treatments that provide diminishing returns. Structural correction interrupts this cycle by addressing the root cause of visible aging.

The psychological and emotional impact of structural rejuvenation extends beyond appearance alone. Facial aging often creates a disconnect between how patients feel internally and how they believe they are perceived externally. This misalignment can affect confidence, social engagement, and professional interactions.

By restoring facial structure in a natural and durable way, the DeepFrame Facelift™ often realigns internal and external identity. Patients describe feeling more confident and comfortable in social settings. Because the result is recognizable and not overtly surgical, this confidence feels authentic rather than performative.

Importantly, this psychological adaptation tends to be stable over time. Because the face continues to age naturally rather than abruptly reverting, patients do not experience the disappointment that can accompany early relapse after superficial procedures. Satisfaction is reinforced rather than eroded as years pass.

Comparisons with non structural interventions frequently arise during long term follow up. Patients who have experienced both approaches often describe a qualitative difference that extends beyond degree of improvement. Rather than chasing individual features such as folds, hollows, or laxity, structural correction produces a sense of overall balance and completeness.

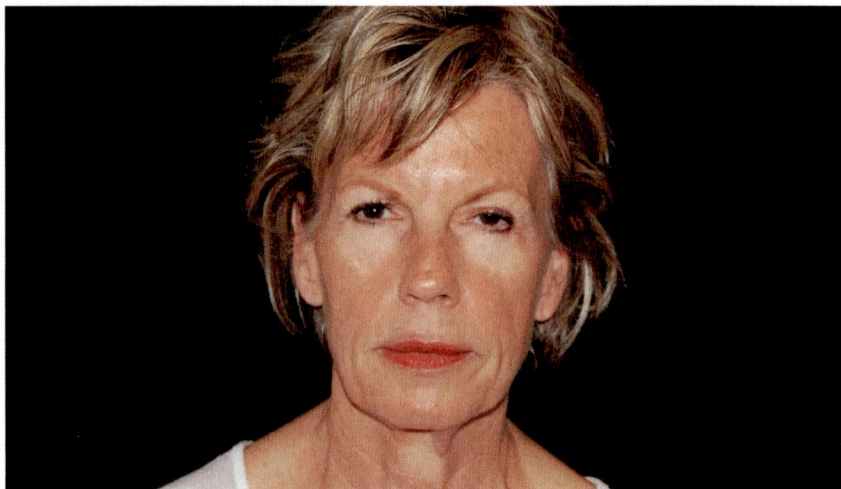

The DeepFrame Facelift™ provides identity
preservation while aligning psychological age with
external appearance.

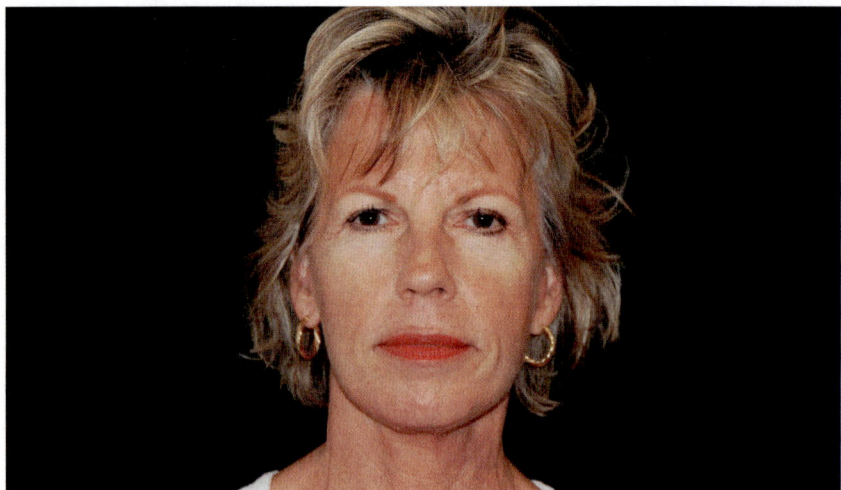

This distinction reinforces the conceptual advantage of addressing aging as a system. When anatomy is restored, surface features improve as a consequence rather than as isolated targets. Patients often express relief at no longer needing to analyze their face in segments or plan serial treatments to maintain appearance.

Long term follow up after structural facelift surgery also shapes the patient surgeon relationship. Because the foundation is stable, follow up focuses on monitoring rather than correction. Visits emphasize assessment of aging progression, skin quality, and patient goals rather than troubleshooting recurrent deformities.

This relationship is collaborative rather than reactive. Adjunctive treatments are discussed in the context of maintenance rather than repair. Patients feel supported over time, and trust is reinforced by the durability and natural evolution of their result.

From a broader perspective, outcomes after the DeepFrame Facelift™ reflect the alignment of surgical philosophy with patient priorities. Most patients do not seek dramatic alteration. They seek restoration, confidence, and longevity. They want to look like themselves, only less burdened by the visible effects of aging.

Structural rejuvenation addresses these priorities directly. By restoring deep anatomical relationships, it produces durable harmony rather than transient improvement. By preserving identity and function, it supports psychological well being. By aging gracefully rather than abruptly, it sustains satisfaction over time.

In this sense, outcomes are not defined by a single endpoint, but by a trajectory. The DeepFrame Facelift™ establishes a favorable trajectory in which the face moves forward through time from a corrected anatomical configuration. This trajectory, rather than any single postoperative moment, is the true measure of success.

Patient satisfaction after structural rejuvenation reflects not only how the face looks, but how it moves, how it ages, and how it feels to inhabit. These dimensions are inseparable. By addressing them collectively, the DeepFrame approach positions itself not simply as a facelift technique, but as a comprehensive framework for long term facial rejuvenation and patient experience.

CHAPTER 15

The DeepFrame Facelift™ as an Evolving Framework for Structural Facial Rejuvenation

Facial rejuvenation has never been static. It has advanced in parallel with deeper anatomical understanding, improved surgical safety, and a growing recognition that youthful appearance is governed less by the condition of the skin than by the integrity of the structures beneath it. The DeepFrame Facelift™ reflects this progression by positioning facelift surgery not as a finite technique, but as a flexible, anatomy driven framework. Its significance lies not only in what it accomplishes today, but in how it accommodates future refinement as knowledge, technology, and patient expectations continue to evolve.

This concluding chapter places the DeepFrame approach within the broader arc of facial rejuvenation and clarifies its role as a living system rather than a fixed procedure. It represents a synthesis of anatomical insight, biomechanical reasoning, and surgical judgment, all organized around the goal of restoring facial structure in a way that is natural, durable, and respectful of individual identity.

Historically, the evolution of facelift surgery has been marked by a series of incremental solutions to clearly defined problems. Early skin based lifts addressed visible laxity but failed to account for relapse and distortion. SMAS based techniques improved durability but often treated the face as a uniform mechanical sheet. Deep plane approaches advanced the concept of composite tissue mobilization, yet frequently relied on relatively fixed vectors and limited regional differentiation. Each phase represented progress, but each also revealed the limitations of focusing on isolated layers or maneuvers.

The DeepFrame Facelift™ represents a conceptual shift away from technique based thinking toward systems based reasoning. Facial aging is understood as a multilevel process involving skeletal remodeling, displacement of deep fat compartments, attenuation of retaining ligaments, elongation of fascial support, and secondary changes in skin.[3-5] These processes do not occur independently. They interact across facial regions, redistributing load and altering spatial relationships over time. Effective rejuvenation must therefore address the face as a coordinated structural system rather than as a collection of discrete problems.

Within this framework, surgical decision making is organized around anatomy and biomechanics rather than procedural checklists. The depth of correction is matched to the depth of pathology. Vectors are selected based on the direction of tissue descent rather than convenience of access. Facial regions are treated in relation to one another rather than in isolation. This orientation allows the procedure to remain conceptually consistent while being technically adaptable.

One of the defining strengths of the DeepFrame Facelift™ is its capacity to incorporate emerging anatomical knowledge without abandoning its foundational principles. Ongoing research continues to refine understanding of facial fat compartment behavior, skeletal change over time, and the mechanical properties of fascia and ligamentous structures. Advances in imaging and long term outcome analysis further clarify how tissues respond to surgical repositioning and how aging resumes after correction.

Because the DeepFrame approach is grounded in structural relationships rather than proprietary tools or singular techniques, it can evolve alongside these insights. Adjustments in how midface elevation is optimized, how SMAS manipulation is tailored, or how cervical support is reinforced can be integrated within the existing framework. This adaptability ensures that the approach remains relevant as understanding deepens, rather than becoming obsolete as techniques change.

The same adaptability applies to integration with adjunctive technologies. Modern aesthetic practice includes a wide array of non surgical and minimally invasive modalities, including resurfacing techniques, neuromodulators, regenerative therapies, and energy based devices. These tools are often promoted as alternatives to surgery, yet their effectiveness is frequently limited when underlying structural displacement remains uncorrected.

Within the DeepFrame framework, adjunctive technologies are positioned as complements rather than substitutes. Structural correction establishes the anatomical foundation upon which surface treatments can be applied more effectively and with greater longevity. Skin quality can be improved without compensating for laxity. Neuromodulators can refine expression without masking imbalance. Regenerative therapies can enhance tissue health within a restored anatomical environment. This sequencing reduces reliance on repetitive interventions and aligns each modality with its appropriate role.

As new technologies emerge, their value can be assessed in relation to restored anatomy rather than as isolated solutions. This perspective encourages thoughtful integration rather than indiscriminate adoption and reinforces the primacy of structure in long term facial rejuvenation.

The DeepFrame Facelift™ also carries important implications for surgical education and professional development. Because the approach emphasizes anatomical reasoning, three dimensional thinking, and intraoperative judgment, it resists commoditization. It cannot be reduced to a standardized protocol or delegated to rote execution. Mastery requires deep familiarity with facial anatomy, comfort with multiple planes of dissection, and the ability to adapt strategy based on real time tissue behavior.

Training within this framework prioritizes understanding over memorization. Surgeons are encouraged to think in terms of load distribution, vector alignment, and structural continuity rather than isolated maneuvers. This mode of thinking extends beyond facelift surgery itself and informs broader aesthetic practice. Surgeons trained to reason structurally are better equipped to evaluate new techniques critically, to individualize care responsibly, and to maintain consistency of outcome across diverse patient populations.

From the patient perspective, the DeepFrame Facelift™ provides a clearer and more intuitive explanation of why certain deep plane approaches produce more durable and natural results. Patients increasingly seek authenticity, longevity, and preservation of identity. A structural framework allows these goals to be articulated in concrete terms. Aging is explained as displacement rather than deficiency. Surgery is framed as restoration rather than alteration. Expectations are aligned with biology rather than marketing.

This shared understanding strengthens the patient surgeon relationship. Patients are better equipped to make informed decisions and to appreciate the value of comprehensive correction over incremental camouflage. Satisfaction is reinforced not only by outcome, but also by understanding the rationale behind it.

At its core, the DeepFrame Facelift™ represents a philosophy of care as much as a surgical approach. It prioritizes anatomy over appearance, restoration over manipulation, and durability over immediacy. It recognizes the face as a living, dynamic system whose integrity depends on the relationships among its components. This philosophy influences how aging is assessed, how interventions are sequenced, and how success is defined.

Rather than attempting to halt aging or impose an idealized aesthetic, the DeepFrame approach seeks to recalibrate anatomy so that aging resumes from a healthier and more balanced configuration. This perspective aligns surgical intervention with the natural biology of the face and supports outcomes that remain satisfying as time passes.

The enduring value of the DeepFrame Facelift™ lies in its flexibility. It is not a destination, but a framework within which facial rejuvenation can continue to evolve. As anatomical understanding advances and patient priorities shift, the principles of deep structural restoration, regional integration, and biomechanical efficiency remain applicable.

By grounding facial rejuvenation in anatomy and systems based thinking, the DeepFrame approach offers a durable foundation for current practice and future innovation. Its contribution is not limited to a single technique, but extends to how surgeons think about aging, how patients understand their options, and how the field continues to refine the art and science of facial rejuvenation.

Appendix A: References

1.   Rohrich RJ, Pessa JE. The fat compartments of the face: anatomy and clinical implications for cosmetic surgery. Plast Reconstr Surg. 2007;119(7):2219-2227.

2.   Gierloff M, Stöhring C, Buder T, Gassling V, Acil Y, Wiltfang J. Aging changes of the midfacial fat compartments: a computed tomographic study. Plast Reconstr Surg. 2012;129(1):263-273.

3.   Mendelson B, Wong CH. Anatomy of the aging face. Clin Plast Surg. 2016;43(3):371-384.

4.   Shaw RB Jr, Katzel EB, Koltz PF, et al. Aging of the midface skeletal elements: a three-dimensional computed tomographic study. Plast Reconstr Surg. 2011;127(1):204-213.

5.   Stuzin JM, Baker TJ, Gordon HL. The relationship of the superficial and deep facial fascia: relevance to rhytidectomy. Plast Reconstr Surg. 1992;89(3):441-449.

6.   Furnas DW. The retaining ligaments of the cheek. Plast Reconstr Surg. 1989;83(1):11-16.

7.   Hamra ST. The deep-plane rhytidectomy. Plast Reconstr Surg. 1990;86(1):53-61.

8.   Stuzin JM. The anatomy and clinical application of the deep plane facelift. Clin Plast Surg. 2018;45(3):229-249.

9.   Marten TJ. High SMAS facelift: combined SMAS plication and deep-plane

elevation. Plast Reconstr Surg. 2008;121(6):2025-2037.

10.   Ramirez OM. Subperiosteal rhytidectomy: the subperiosteal facelift. Plast Reconstr Surg. 1992;90(3):367-378.

11.   Little JW. Volumetric rejuvenation of the aging midface with subperiosteal elevation. Aesthetic Surg J. 2000;20(2):137-142.

12.   Barton FE Jr. The tear trough deformity: an anatomical perspective. Plast Reconstr Surg. 1992;89(3):430-435.

13.   Goldberg RA, McCann JD, Fiaschetti D, Ben Simon GJ. What causes eyelid bags? Analysis of 114 consecutive patients. Plast Reconstr Surg. 2005;115(5):1395-1402.

14.   Mendelson BC. Facelift anatomy, SMAS, retaining ligaments and facial spaces. Aesthetic Surg J. 2012;32(5):578-593.

15.   Rohrich RJ, Pessa JE. The retaining system of the face: histologic evaluation of the septal boundaries of the facial fat compartments. Plast Reconstr Surg. 2008;121(5):1804-1809.

16.   Rauso R, Salti G, Zerbinati N. Complications of facial fillers: an update. J Cosmet Dermatol. 2020;19(8):1873-1881.

17.   American Society for Aesthetic Plastic Surgery. Facial filler complications: safety review. Aesthetic Surg J. 2021;41(4):NP391-NP403.9. Owsley JQ Jr. SMAS-platysma face lift. Plast Reconstr Surg. 1978;61(4):517-523. doi:10.1097/00006534-197804000-00001

18.   Feldman JJ. Neck lift classification system. Plast Reconstr Surg. 2014;134(2):287–297.

19.   Stuzin JM, Baker TJ. Cervicofacial anatomy and the SMAS–platysma complex. Clin Plast Surg. 2018;45(3):265–276.

20.   Mendelson BC, Muzaffar AR. The superficial fascia of the neck and face. Plast Reconstr Surg. 2002;109(2):707–720.

21.   Pessa JE, Zadoo VP, Mutimer KL, et al. Relative maxillary and mandibular aging and its clinical relevance. Plast Reconstr Surg. 1998;102(1):205–212.

22.   Owsley JQ, Agarwal CA. SMAS facelift: a 20-year experience. Plast Reconstr Surg. 2008;121(6):2197–2207.

23.   Truswell WH. Longevity of the deep-plane facelift. Aesthetic Surg J. 2015;35(4):411–418.

24.   Marten TJ. Facelift longevity: what lasts and why. Clin Plast Surg. 2013;40(4):625–636.

25.   Rohrich RJ, Ghavami A. Avoiding unnatural results in facelift surgery. Plast Reconstr Surg. 2009;124(3):1393–1404.

26.   Jacono AA, Malone MH. Revision facelift surgery. Facial Plast Surg Clin North Am. 2019;27(3):353–364.

27.   Stuzin JM. Face lifting. In: Neligan PC, ed. Plastic Surgery. 4th ed. Elsevier; 2018:193–223.

28.	Mendelson BC. Systematic facial rejuvenation. Aesthetic Plast Surg. 2010;34(4):411–420.

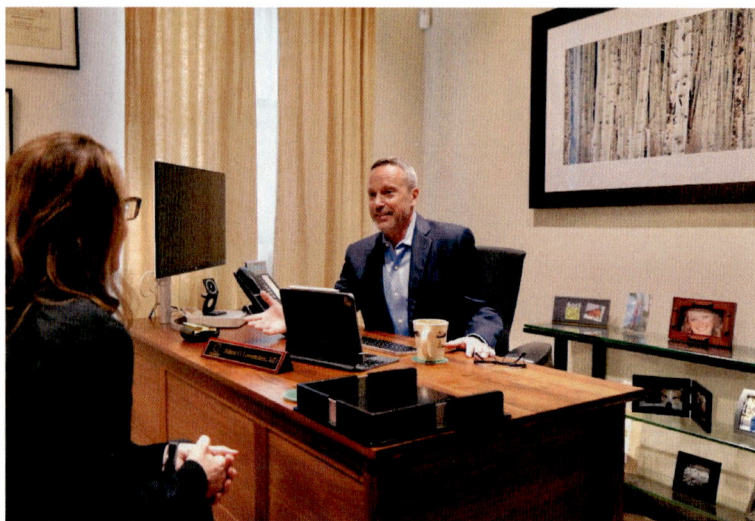

About the Author: Adam Lowenstein, MD

Adam Lowenstein, MD, is a board-certified plastic surgeon and the creator of the DeepFrame Facelift™, a structural, anatomy-based facial rejuvenation system that integrates sub-periosteal midface elevation, multi-vector SMAS and platysma manipulation, and continuous deep-plane mobilization across the midface, lower face, jawline, and neck.

He specializes in advanced facelift surgery and peripheral nerve decompression surgery for chronic headaches, combining more than twenty years of surgical experience with a deep and evolving understanding of facial and cranial anatomy.

Dr. Lowenstein has been double boarded in both General Surgery and Plastic Surgery. He was trained in general surgery at Thomas Jefferson University in Philadelphia and plastic surgery at the University of Massachusetts, followed by a career that spans both aesthetic and reconstructive disciplines. His early work in reconstructive microsurgery provided a foundation in three-dimensional anatomical relationships, tissue biomechanics, and surgical precision- skills that ultimately shaped the development of the DeepFrame Facelift™. After relocating to Santa Barbara, he focused his practice on aesthetic facial surgery and headache surgery, earning a reputation for natural, identity-preserving outcomes and a structural, evidence-based approach to rejuvenation.

In addition to his facial surgery practice, Dr. Lowenstein is one of the nation's most experienced surgeons in nerve decompression surgery for chronic headaches and is the author of *Headache Surgery: Understanding a Path Forward*. His work in both fields is grounded in a commitment to scientific clarity, patient education, and surgical innovation.

Dr. Lowenstein is the creator and primary authority on the DeepFrame Facelift™, a structural facelift system that originated from his two decades of surgical experience and anatomical research. His academic interests include facial aging biomechanics, midface and cervicofacial anatomy, deep-plane surgical technique evolution, and the psychology of identity preservation in aesthetic surgery.

He lives in Santa Barbara with his wife and children.

Made in the USA
Las Vegas, NV
25 January 2026

40239578R10112